Lifestyle in Medicine

In western societies, 'lifestyle' as an explanation for health and illness has become increasingly popular. Certain concepts of lifestyle are now at the fore in epidemiology, public health and preventive medicine and as such we are constantly being told that we should not smoke, overeat, drink too much or exercise too little. This emphasis on social factors has led to the assertion that we are responsible for our own health, but to what extent is this true?

Lifestyle in Medicine explores the ambiguity of the term 'lifestyle' and the way it is conceived and applied within medicine. Based on real doctor/patient consultations and in-depth interviews with doctors, the book discusses:

- the history behind current medical use of lifestyle
- the variable usage of the 'lifestyle' concept in different medical settings
- critical writings and recent shifts in sociological thinking about lifestyle
- public and government concerns about unhealthy lifestyles
- the ways in which health is discussed, doctor to patient.

Evidence-based in its approach, *Lifestyle in Medicine* uses original research to highlight this topical issue and provides professional and lay perspectives on health and illness. It is essential reading for students and academics of medical sociology, health and allied health studies and anyone interested in health and society.

Emily Hansen is Research Fellow in primary health care research at the University of Tasmania, Australia.

Gary Easthope is Reader in Sociology at the University of Tasmania, Australia.

Critical studies in health and society
Edited by Simon J. Williams and Gillian Bendelow

This major new international book series takes a critical look at health in a rapidly changing social world. The series includes theoretically sophisticated and empirically informed contributions on cutting-edge issues from leading figures within the sociology of health and allied disciplines and domains. Other titles in the series include:

Contesting Psychiatry
Social movements in mental health
Nick Crossley

Men and their Health
Masculinity, social inequality and health
Alan Dolan

Lifestyle in Medicine
Emily Hansen and Gary Easthope

Medical Sociology and Old Age
Towards a sociology of health in later life
Paul Higgs and Ian Rees Jones

Emotional Labour in Health Care
Catherine Theodosius

Written in a lively, accessible and engaging style, with many thought-provoking insights, the series caters to a truly interdisciplinary audience of researchers, professionals, practitioners and policy makers with an interest in health and social change.

Those interested in submitting proposals for single or co-authored, edited or co-edited volumes should contact the series editors, Simon J. Williams (s.j.williams@warwick.ac.uk) and Gillian Bendelow (g.a.bendelow@sussex.ac.uk).

Lifestyle in Medicine

Emily Hansen and Gary Easthope

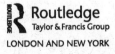
Routledge
Taylor & Francis Group

LONDON AND NEW YORK

First published 2007 by Routledge
4 Park Square, Milton Park, Abingdon, Oxon OX14 4RN
605 Third Avenue, New York, NY 10017

Routledge is an imprint of the Taylor & Francis Group, an informa business

© 2007 Emily Hansen and Gary Easthope

Typeset in Sabon by RefineCatch Limited, Bungay, Suffolk

British Library Cataloguing in Publication Data
A catalogue record for this book is available from the British Library

Library of Congress Cataloging in Publication Data
A catalog record for this book has been requested

ISBN13: 978-0-415-35684-8 (hbk)
ISBN13: 978-0-415-35685-5 (pbk)
ISBN13: 978-0-203-00284-1 (ebk)

Contents

Preface

This monograph is a reflection upon the concept of lifestyle as it is used in medicine and sociology. Lifestyle, as will become clear, is not a simple concept. Through examining its complexity we are able to gain insight into the complexity of medical life and the boundary issues that arise between medicine and sociology.

This reflection was produced over several years in a dialogue between the two authors. The first author, Emily, began the dialogue as a doctoral student supervised by the second author, Gary. This dialogue was conducted during supervisory meetings, monthly seminars at Gary's house and innumerable hallway debates. The book draws heavily on Emily's doctoral thesis and the empirical work she did for it. This is most obvious in the chapters that report the empirical work (chapters 4 and 5) and we denote it in the text by using 'Emily', rather than 'we', the authors, in those chapters. However, the dialogue did not cease upon completion of the thesis. Both authors continued their work together as colleagues rather than supervisor and student. Neither did sociologists cease to write about lifestyle nor lifestyle shift from a central position in public health policies and funded research.

However, the thesis lies at its core and thus the book should be read as the work of Emily Hansen conducted with the assistance of her one-time supervisor and now colleague, Gary Easthope.

Acknowledgements

We owe thanks to many people who assisted us while we were writing this book.

To Dr Chris Easthope who not only provided food for the body in those many evening seminars but also contributed to the dialogue.

To Rita Johnson, Joel Stafford, Margaret Hansen and Paul Hansen, all of whom supported Emily during the writing of the thesis and this book.

Thank you to all of the research participants, our colleagues in the School of Sociology and Social Work and the Discipline of General Practice at the University of Tasmania, and all others who assisted us with the research including Della Clark and Lyn Devereaux.

Finally Emily would like to acknowledge salary support from the Australian Commonwealth Department of Health and Aging via the Primary Health Care Research Evaluation and Development Strategy Research Capacity Building Initiative (PHCRED).

Introduction

Let us start by asking you, the reader, a few simple questions about your lifestyle and health. We want you to be honest in your answers to yourself. Nobody else need know what you reply. Just answer yes or no.

Are you too fat? Do you smoke? Do you drink too much? Are you physically inactive?

If you answered yes to any of those questions do you feel guilty about it? If you answered no to any of them do you feel smugly superior?

If you feel either guilty or superior – and we are confident you will feel one or the other – you are responding to the fact that aspects of your lifestyle (your eating, smoking, drinking and exercising) are seen by you as good or bad for your health. You are seeing these actions or states as health related and you are making a moral judgement about your own behaviour. It is also very possible that you feel there is something intrinsically unhealthy about contemporary western lifestyles.

This is not surprising. You, just like us – the authors – and everyone else in modern societies, are constantly bombarded with messages that if you want to keep healthy you should do certain things. You should (note the moral imperative command 'should') not smoke, you should not overeat, you should drink alcohol in moderation and you should take exercise. Further, it is expected that you should (again should) keep healthy.

The final three decades of the twentieth century saw certain concepts of lifestyle brought to the fore in the fields of epidemiology, public health and health promotion. Some writers suggest that by the mid-1990s lifestyle and associated notions about behavioural risk factors had become the dominant medical explanatory concept (Hughes 1994; Petersen and Lupton 1996). Lifestyle also became a buzzword in the popular media, complementary and alternative medicine, allied health and general practice (Crawford 1978, 1980; Fitzgerald 1994; Petersen 1996). The increasing popularity of lifestyle as an explanatory concept in the late twentieth century is recognised as an important shift within popular conceptions of health (e.g. Crawford 1978, 1980; Featherstone 1987; Blaxter 1990; White *et al.* 1995), within health-related policies at national and international levels (Ashton and Seymour 1988; Bunton and Macdonald 1992), and within medical thought in general (Davies 1984; Hughes 1994; Armstrong 1995; Labonte 1995).

However, the relationship between lifestyle factors and people's health and even the meaning of lifestyle as a term remain ambiguous (Coreil *et al.* 1985; Davison and Davey Smith 1995). Despite all the effort to promote a healthy lifestyle it is not clear what constitutes a healthy lifestyle or whether or not adopting one will result in disease prevention or increased longevity. Concern about this has resulted in a plethora of research and lifestyle-related popular cultural forms such as self-help books, advice columns and the ultimate social barometers, jokes. For example:

> The Japanese eat little fat and suffer fewer heart attacks than Australians or New Zealanders. The French eat a lot of fat and also suffer fewer heart attacks than Australians or New Zealanders. The Italians drink a lot of red wine and also suffer fewer heart attacks than Australians or New Zealanders.
>   Conclusion: eat and drink what you like. Speaking English is what kills you.
>   *Irwin Knopf*
> (*Australian Readers Digest* November 2002: 73)

Despite the vast amounts of research investigating statistical relationships between lifestyle factors and disease very little is known about the way medicine in general or doctors in particular talk about lifestyle or apply concepts related to it when explaining health and illness.

To remedy that lack of knowledge about medical understandings of lifestyle we draw together in this book what is known about such understandings and report on our empirical research on the topic. In short, the book explores the way that lifestyle is conceived and applied within medicine. In it we address a number of unanswered questions about medical understandings of lifestyle. As sociologists we have an intrinsic interest in medical attempts to construct and apply a social model of disease (Becker 1993). However, we also wish to address the relative neglect of medical explanatory frameworks by sociologists when compared to the large body of investigation into lay understandings of health and disease. We wish in this way to contribute significantly to the body of sociological writing which expresses concern about many aspects of medical understandings of lifestyle in the context of a wider critique of contemporary public health practices and ideologies (e.g. Crawford 1978, 1980; Castel 1991; Armstrong 1993, 1995; Fitzgerald 1994; Duff 1999).

This writing has been largely focused on how lifestyle is understood in epidemiological research into social determinants or 'risk factors' for disease and in epidemiologically driven public health. As the popularity and influence of those forms of epidemiology and public health that focused on lifestyle modification grew throughout the 1980s and early 1990s, so too did this body of sociological literature. By the mid-1990s sociological writing critical of a lifestyle approach had become the new sociological orthodoxy on this subject.

We consider there are several areas of underdevelopment in sociological knowledge about medical understandings of lifestyle that suggest a need for additional research. First, many sociologists have taken at face value the idea that there is one notion of lifestyle held by medicine. Sociological writers criticising the ways that lifestyle is used within medicine as an explanatory framework have focused almost entirely on epidemiology or public health. This leaves us ignorant about how individual doctors construct and apply ideas about lifestyle and how lifestyle might be understood and applied in fields other than epidemiology and public health. While approaching medicine as a unified collective is integral to a critical sociological perspective, which by its nature necessitates a concrete and stable object, it is also problematic in the context of sociological and anthropological debate about medical knowledge. This raises the strong possibility that medical knowledge is not homogeneous or unified, but instead, should be understood as heterogeneous, contextual and fragmented (Helman 1978, 1981a, 1981b, 1985a, 1988; Gordon 1988a; Gaines and Hahn 1985; Fox 1993; Atkinson 1995).

It is also problematic in the context of a long-recognised medical differentiation between and within the fields of epidemiology, public health and mainstream medicine. Epidemiologists and medical doctors are trained differently. Epidemiologists are not necessarily trained medical doctors; they are equally likely to be specialists in the fields of population health, statistics, scientific research and demography. Many medical schools offer little or no epidemiology in their undergraduate courses. Public health is a paramedical discipline which, although primarily biomedical in outlook, is historically and practically distinct from mainstream medicine. Within the fields of epidemiology and public health, lifestyle arguments are only some of the many different models of disease and health in use.

Furthermore, focusing on the fields of epidemiology and public health and criticising an abstract, unified medicine has resulted in the understandings of individual doctors about lifestyle, health and disease being taken as *given*. In the same way that the traditional sociological distinction between disease and illness left doctors' understandings unexplored by sociologists because they were assumed to be stable and objective, conflating medical understandings of lifestyle with representations of epidemiological or public health understandings serves to erase the possibility that medical understandings of lifestyle might be complex because they are assumed to be self-evident. As argued by Strong (1979a) and Williams (2001), the various disciplines that make up medicine are not unified in their theories, their science or their methods. Thus sociologists should not take evidence from one part of medicine and use it to argue about the nature of medicine as a whole.

Focusing on epidemiology and public health has also resulted in lifestyle models being seen only as *preventive models*. If as Hughes (1994) and Petersen and Lupton (1996) consider, a lifestyle approach is becoming the predominant explanatory framework within medicine, then it seems probable that lifestyle understandings would not be limited in their application to preventive contexts. Doctors are not only concerned with disease, but must also account for health and illness. In addition to disease prevention, medical practice involves data gathering, investigation, diagnosis, treatment of acute disorders and management of chronic ones (Gammon 1990). While lifestyle arguments might have originated in the context of the prevention of disease, like other medical models of disease they are not bound to their original context and may well transcend it.

This issue, of how lifestyle understandings of health and disease are actually constructed, interpreted and applied by medical doctors, is an important one. How understandings of lifestyle are used by doctors (as an explanatory framework) to deal with 'real' illnesses requires investigation. The clinical application of a lifestyle perspective has been inferred, and only rarely investigated by sociologists.

The next issue requiring further sociological investigation is the relationship between medical and lay perspectives on lifestyle. In the sociological literature it has been usual for writers to consider lay and medical understandings to be quite distinct. In much of the sociological literature patients have 'folk illnesses' and construct 'explanatory models' while doctors deal with 'disease entities' and 'medical facts' (Prior *et al.* 2000). However, empirical research has blurred this distinction by demonstrating that doctors also construct their own explanatory models to make sense of situations and that these models utilise folk, commonsense and personal knowledges in addition to specialised scientific medical knowledges (e.g. Helman 1981a, 1981b, 1988; Gaines and Hahn 1985).

However, lay and medical understandings of lifestyle have often been treated as distinct and separate knowledges (e.g. Blaxter 1990; Pierret 1993; Backett and Davison 1995). Lay understandings of lifestyle have been represented as being folk or commonsense understandings of health and illness (Pill 1991; Popay *et al.* 1998), or as being developed in conjunction with, in reaction to, or in opposition to medical understandings (e.g. Blaxter 1997; Smith 1998). Medical understandings have generally been treated as being stable, easily identifiable as 'medical', and a point of reference to which lay understandings can be compared (e.g. Davison *et al.* 1991, 1992; Frankel *et al.* 1991).

The sociological distinction between lay and medical knowledge perpetuated in sociological writing about lifestyle has excluded doctors from the processes of lay knowledge construction about lifestyle. However, doctors are not isolated entities; they are community members and as such are not excluded from lay processes of knowledge construction (Helman 1985a, 1985b; Good 1994; Atkinson 1995). Expert knowledge among doctors cannot be assumed when investigating understandings of disease that rely heavily on epidemiological models. These are highly specialised and esoteric. Without epidemiological training most doctors are unlikely to have the statistical knowledge to fully understand epidemiological models of risk and lifestyle. In this situation many doctors should not be considered as scientific experts in the field of epidemiology and population health. Instead, they are in a similar situation to well-educated non-medical people who utilise understandings of lifestyle, and interpretations of epidemiological models of risk in particular, which they have acquired from other sources. These sources, such as health promotion material, practitioner education in disease prevention and the popular press are not strictly 'medical' knowledges.

The assumption that medical understandings of lifestyle are predictable and distinct from lay understandings of lifestyle is also ironic in the light of continued sociological comments that lifestyle risk factor approaches to explaining disease are moralistic and discriminatory precisely because they reflect and reproduce so many sociocultural notions (Crawford 1978, 1980; Hughes 1994; Vertinsky 1998; Williams 1998). If doctors' understandings of lifestyle are assumed not to be restricted to epidemiological and public health understandings but perhaps also to include lay notions of lifestyle, then medical understandings of lifestyle are likely to be far more complex and multi-faceted than has previously been supposed in the sociological literature. They may also be quite different from sociological characterisations of medical understandings of lifestyle. For example, Lupton (1993), Hughes (1994) and Petersen (1996) have all pointed to the moralistic nature of medical understandings of lifestyle. Studies show that lay people reject the aspects of public health lifestyle explanations that imply that individuals are responsible for their illness. Instead, they accept the argument that a 'healthy' lifestyle results in good health and explain poor health in terms of bad luck, chance or individual susceptibility (Davison *et al.* 1991, 1992). If doctors integrate lay conceptions of lifestyle when they construct their own understandings, these may include a reluctance to explain disease in terms of lifestyle in a moralistic fashion.

Lifestyle-focused explanatory frameworks are very open to the inclusion of folk and commonsense knowledges because they refer to everyday practices and behaviours, utilise everyday language and terms and have been highly popularised through health promotion campaigns. Because of this, they are a perfect site within medical knowledge to explore the relationship between lay and medical knowledge. We view medical understandings of lifestyle as an exciting opportunity to learn more about the processes whereby medical doctors accomplish the construction and utilisation of a dynamic and changeable 'knowledge in practice'.

Because of this we conducted empirical research aiming to explore medical understandings of lifestyle. The book is organised into six chapters. The first chapter describes the complexity of medical understandings of disease. Medical explanatory frameworks focusing on lifestyle are described and located historically and in relation to other medical frameworks used by doctors to explain disease. They are also discussed in relation to wider social processes of late/high modernity, demographic changes associated with advanced capitalist societies and government policies on public health. Medical and lay understandings of lifestyle are compared.

In chapter 2 we present the first aspect of the sociological critique of lifestyle as a medical explanatory framework. This chapter describes how sociologists were originally excited by signs that medical people were utilising a social model of disease. However, differences between sociological and epidemiological/public health ideas about the meaning of lifestyle and the relationship between individual lifestyles and disease led to reductive understandings of disease with only limited efficacy for preventing disease or improving health outcomes. To support this claim we present convincing evidence drawn from public health and epidemiology showing that programmes aiming to prevent disease by modifying people's lifestyle have been a resounding failure in a number of different countries.

Chapter 3 presents a sociocultural critique of 'lifestylism', risk factor epidemiology and lifestyle-focused health promotion. In this chapter we describe the assumptions underpinning a lifestyle approach to disease and draw on a number of sociological writers to outline negative implications arising from these. Contemporary medical understandings of lifestyle, health and disease have attracted sociological interest and critique because these ideas have a range of important implications both for those who are being understood and for those who are striving to understand. As a medical explanatory framework, lifestyle is heavily laden with cultural baggage. The most frequently described of these cultural burdens are that lifestyle understandings are moralistic and discriminatory, that they increase the potential for medicalisation, medical surveillance and medical control, that they reflect, reinforce and reproduce contemporary concerns with the management and containment of risks, that they are associated with commodifying and commercialising the body and health and that they are modernist and science based. The chapter concludes with three research questions that form the basis of the empirical research presented in the remaining chapters of the book.

In chapter 4 we present the results of a thematic review of medical and lay texts, and describe the range of different ways that lifestyle is conceptualised within them. These texts are presented as a typology of different medical and lay conceptions of lifestyle. Chapter 5 presents evidence from in-depth interviews with doctors, observation of doctor/patient consultations and participant observation of doctor/patient consultations to describe six different ways that doctors explain health, illness and disease in terms of lifestyle. Chapter 6 provides an overview of the results. They are discussed in relation to the sociological critique of lifestyle as a medical explanatory framework and wider theoretical issues for medical sociology/sociology of health and illness. We also discuss the results in the light of changes that occurred in the years since our empirical research was completed and reflect on the future of lifestyle as a medical explanatory approach.

1   Lifestyle as a medical explanatory model

Introduction

This chapter begins our exploration of the concept of lifestyle as a medical explanatory model. In it we describe the ways that disease is explained in contemporary western medicine and draw attention to the differences between the traditional biomedical model and a social lifestyle model of disease. We trace the emergence of lifestyle as a medical concept and link this emergence with a number of social processes and the increasing role played by epidemiology as a medically legitimate source of knowledge. Medical understandings of lifestyle are very interesting because they raise a number of issues of importance such as the usefulness of traditional sociological characterisations of medical knowledge and practice (the disease/illness distinction, the medical model, the medical/lay dichotomy); the emergence of a lifestyle model of disease; links between wider social processes and medical knowledge; the increasing prominence of epidemiology in the latter half of the twentieth century and differences and similarities between expert and lay knowledges about health and disease.

Medical models and medical explanations for disease

To the medical doctor, explanation refers to diagnosis, providing the disorder with a name and identifying symptoms or proximal causes (Open University 1985). The standard medical approach to explaining sickness is usually represented as a continuously developing, coherent one which, through scientific research, is able to uncover the truth about the 'real', that is biological, determinants of disease (Temkin 1981). This approach has been described as the 'medical model' or the 'biomedical model' (Atkinson 1988: 180). The phrase medical model is used interchangeably to describe two different models. First, the term is used to describe the pre-eminent scientific model used by those involved with medical science for the explanation of disease. For the sake of clarity we will refer to this as the medical model. However, the term is also used to describe a sociological 'ideal type' constructed to describe the medical approach to disease. This ideal type is based on the assumption that the medical orientation towards disease will be a direct reflection of dominant medical theory.

> The medical model in the medical explanation of disease has a number of important features. Disease is regarded as the consequence of certain malfunctions of the human body conceptualised as a biochemical machine. Secondly, the medical model assumes that all human dysfunctions might eventually be traced to such specific causal mechanisms within the organism; eventually various forms of mental illness would be explicable directly in terms of biochemical changes. The medical model is reductionist in the sense that all disease and illness behaviours would be reduced causally to a number of specific biochemical mechanisms. Furthermore, the medical model is exclusionary in that alternative perspectives would be removed as invalid. Finally the medical model presupposes a clear mind/body distinction where ultimately the causal agent of illness would be located in the human body.
>
> (Turner 1987: 9)

For the sake of clarity we will refer to this as the sociological medical model. As a scientific model of disease, the medical model is primarily based on germ theory (the doctrine of specific aetiology). Germ theory has maintained considerable popularity with policy makers, those working in medicine and the lay public since its inception in the late nineteenth century (Calnan and Williams 1992). The major reason for this popularity is that germ theory (like all scientific and other knowledges) is pervaded by the value systems of late nineteenth- and twentieth-century western societies (Lock 1988). Two of these values are 'naturalism' (that science confers legitimacy and status, and is a universal framework because scientific knowledge is a reflection of an independent empirical reality) and individualism ('a complex of values and assumptions asserting the primacy of the individual and individual freedom' (Gordon 1988a: 21)). Germ theory reflects these values, reinforces them and reproduces them. It is synonymous with science. Furthermore, the methods of disease prevention implied by germ theory do not call for personal change or economic upheaval. Disease outbreaks can be understood as individual instances and disease prevention as a medical responsibility. This has considerable appeal for both policy makers and the lay population. While complex and tangled relationships between disease and the social environment are recognised in germ theory, the real cause of disease is assumed to be tangible, individual and identifiable (Tesh 1990).

As an ideal type within sociology, the sociological medical model has served a number of important functions. It allows for generalisation, comparison and critique and has been an essential aspect of the sociological construction of medicine as 'other' (Atkinson 1995). Furthermore, the sociological medical model implicitly supports and reflects two additional sociological assumptions about the medical approach. These are the medical/lay distinction and the disease/illness distinction.

The medical/lay distinction is the assumption that medical knowledge is easily identified and distinct from lay knowledges about ill-health. In the medical model, medical understandings are associated with surety and scientific logic, and thus implicitly contrasted with lay/folk understandings associated with cultural relativity: 'vagueness, multiplicity of meanings, frequent changes and lack of sharp boundaries between ideas and experience' (Kleinman 1980: 107). This dichotomy is generally expressed in terms of medical knowledge and lay belief (Hahn 1983). In the disease/illness distinction the term disease is used to refer to a natural world of biological processes while the term illness is used to describe social responses to disease (Fabrega 1974; Dingwall 1976; Helman 1985a, 1985b; Bond and Bond 1986).

Thus the concern of medicine is clearly established as the biological cause, nature and treatment of disease while illness is established as the concern of non-medical people, including patients, families and social scientists. Like the sociological medical model, the disease/illness distinction has been a very useful device. In terms of clinical sociology and medical practice, a clearly defined concept of 'illness' has focused much needed attention on the importance of the social, psychological and cultural aspects of disease (Atkinson 1995).

Furthermore, the concept of illness has also provided a standpoint for sociological criticism of the reductive nature of a purely biomechanical conception of ill-health (Dingwall 1976; Calnan 1987). In terms of the development of a theoretical sociology of health and illness, the disease/illness distinction has been a skilled act of boundary maintenance between medicine and sociology, creating a legitimate sphere for sociologists interested in working in the area of health and medicine. By making a theoretical distinction between disease and illness, where disease was conceptualised as biological fact and illness as the social response to disease (primarily that of the person affected by the disease), sociologists were bargaining for space within the primarily medical arena of health and sickness.

However, while the disease and illness distinction, the lay/medical distinction and the medical model describe a particular type of medical approach to disease which is instantly recognisable by both medical and lay people, these descriptors are overly simplistic characterisations of the medical approach to explaining disease. They can only suggest some of the ways that doctors actually account for ill-health. Despite the dominance of germ theory, medicine is characterised by internal diversity rather than internal homogeneity (Strong 1979a, 1979b, 1984; Helman 1985a, 1985b; Lock 1985):

[It is] . . . actually very hard to find this medical model in practice. Few practitioners and no textbooks of any repute subscribe to uni-directional causal models and invariably interventions are seen in medical practice

> as contingent and multi-factorial and ultimately based on assessments and probabilities. Disease taxonomies, aetiologies and therapeutics are used in medical practice as ideal-types, constantly subject to revision . . . medicine tends to be much more holistic than medical sociology traditionally gives it credit for.
>
> (Kelly and Field 1994: 35)

Within medicine there also exists a range of models of disease additional to germ theory. Many of these are in some way able to account for genetics, the environment, the psyche and the social/cultural milieu. Particular variation can be seen between the models used by different types of doctors, for example hospital doctors, private specialists, general practitioners and medical scientists involved in research (Helman 1985a). Different medical specialities emphasise different explanations for disease and health. Thus medical explanations from one area of medicine cannot be taken as synonymous with medical explanations from a different area of medicine (Williams, S. 2001; Strong 1979a).

While these different models, like germ theory, are all science based, individualist, purport to be morally neutral and are frequently interpreted as though they were universally applicable, they also vary between each other and in relation to germ theory. The acceptance and application of environmental, genetic, psychological and lifestyle models within medicine provide pragmatic evidence that medicine is concerned not just with the biological (disease) but also with the social (illness). Furthermore, in the medical model (and the associated disease/illness distinction), disease is a reified entity that is assumed to exist in nature and requires only identification and definition by medical scientists (Hahn 1983). This perspective has been criticised in social constructionist accounts of medical knowledge which argue convincingly that disease as well as illness is a social construct and that all medical understandings, including understandings of disease, are the product of medical discourses which in turn reflect dominant modes of thinking (Wright and Treacher 1982a, 1982b; Nicolson and McLaughlin 1987; Turner 1987; Atkinson 1995).

In addition to a plurality of medically recognised explanatory frameworks for disease, and the issue that scientific knowledge is socially produced and thus inherently imbued with the values and beliefs of the originating culture and time period, the ways that doctors make sense of disease and health are also variable because medical knowledge and practice draw upon 'a background of tacit understandings' that transcend the boundaries of medically accepted and recognised models of disease (Gordon 1988a: 19). Medical knowledge is not only a formalised abstract, theoretical knowledge, but is also knowledge in practice. Therefore, medical knowledge about disease is not static. While it is widely acknowledged that formal medical knowledge will alter over time in response to medical research and changes in social values, it is less widely recognised that at the level of everyday medical practice medical knowledge is in a constant state of flux because it is knowledge in practice (Wright and Treacher 1982b).

At one level this relates to the issue of tacit knowledge formed through experience, the concept of clinical judgement. Physicians learn scientific principles about diagnosis and aetiology which they apply using their own clinical judgement for the purpose of patient care management (Gordon 1988b). Thus formal medical theory will be interpreted and applied in unique ways by the doctors practising medicine. Furthermore, as mentioned above, doctors from different medical disciplines (for example, rheumatology, epidemiology, psychology or general practice) will at times utilise different medically accepted models of disease and interpret these in the manner currently considered legitimate within their field (Siegler 1981). At a second and less widely acknowledged level, medical knowledge and practice are also subject to variability because they are constructed through processes of interaction. The sociological medical model fails to account for the complex processes of interaction that take place during medical work. Helman argues that instead of relying on one model of disease, doctors draw upon a range of different explanatory models (1985b). The term explanatory model is used to describe the understandings that all individuals have about a particular illness episode (Kleinman 1980).

The explanatory model that a doctor constructs to explain a particular episode of ill-health experienced by a patient will be influenced by any of a range of medically accepted models of disease, the doctor's level of medical experience, the identity, views and opinions expressed by that patient and other medical workers, the doctor's life experiences (including observations of their own illnesses and the illnesses of other people) and general beliefs about bodies, health and disease and the situational context (Good and Good 1980; Lock 1985). 'Neither are explanatory models necessarily comprehensive and rigorously coherent; internal contradictions and inconsistencies are common and some elements may be adhered to more strongly than others' (Usherwood 1999: 7).

The day-to-day routines of medical work involve considerable interaction among doctors and between doctors and other medical workers. In a study of haematologists at a large teaching hospital, Atkinson (1995) demonstrated that the construction of medical knowledge about disease (causation, diagnosis, treatment and outcomes) is ongoing and that doctors achieve their medical understandings of it (thus their constructions of explanatory models) not solely on the basis of formalised written medical knowledge but also by talking to each other. This talk occurs in a range of contexts including recurrent cycles of meetings, conferences and informal conversations.

In addition to the interaction that occurs between medical people, there is a complex interrelationship between medical and lay understandings of disease which occurs through interaction during the doctor/patient relationship. This operates at a number of different levels. The descriptions of diagnosis or treatment doctors use when they are talking with their patient are likely to be different from those they use when talking with other doctors. Helman suggests, therefore, that 'one can differentiate between different theoretical models used by physicians but also . . . between these more "scientific" models and the observable clinical ones that they actually employ in their day-to-day practice' (1985a: 294). Over time, a complex interrelationship between doctors' and patients' explanatory models will develop. Patients alter their explanatory models as they are influenced by the models used by their doctor. Equally, doctors alter their explanatory models as they are influenced by their patients' models. 'Each will have a varying amount of influence over the other as diagnosis and treatment take their course' (Helman 1985a: 294).

As can be seen from this discussion of explanatory models and the ways that medical knowledge (including knowledge about disease) is culturally produced, the traditional sociological distinction between lay and medical knowledge is highly problematic. Medical understandings have been shown to be inherently imbued with 'non-scientific' or popular conceptions of health and illness (Gabbay 1982; Helman 1985a, 1985b; Gordon 1988a; Kirmayer 1988) and to be characterised by attributes similar to lay understandings: for example, being changeable, contingent and pluralistic (Good and Good 1980; Gaines and Hahn 1985). Furthermore, studies have demonstrated that lay understandings of disease have many similarities to academic theories of illness and disease in that they demonstrate the application of expertise and frequently include scientific medical knowledge (West 1979; Calnan 1987; Stacey 1988; Whittaker 1995; Popay *et al.* 1998; Prior *et al.* 2000).

In summary, medical explanatory frameworks for disease are not straightforward. The medical model and associated assumptions about the disease/illness distinction and the lay/medical distinction indicate some of the defining characteristics of the medical approach to disease: that it claims legitimacy and methods from science; that it is primarily focused on the biological; that it is a universalistic and individualist framework; and that it is constructed and presented in opposition to other (non-medical/non-scientific) approaches towards disease. Many decades of sociological and anthropological research into medicine have shown that medical explanatory frameworks for disease do contain these elements (Cartwright 1977; Davis and George 1990; Nettleton 1995). Furthermore, these are some of the characteristics by which medicine defines itself (Starr 1982; Willis 1983).

However, the use of the medical model, both by medical writers and by sociologists, operates on the assumption that medicine is a unified, coherent, stable and homogeneous body of knowledge and practice which is clearly distinct from other knowledges about bodies, sickness, health and healing. This is a questionable assumption. Rather, medicine appears to be an institution marked by considerable internal diversity of opinion and practice; medical knowledge is to varying degrees shifting and contingent while the boundaries between medical and non-medical knowledge are ambiguous.

As such, the ways that doctors make sense of disease and health can only be partially described in the medical model and generalisations about any medical approach to disease are likely to conceal complexity and variation.

Lifestyle theories of health and disease

As outlined above, the most widely recognised and probably the most widely used explanatory framework within medicine is germ theory. Germ theory has been the dominant theory of the body and disease within western cultures and medicine since the nineteenth century. Germ theory locates the cause of each specific disease in a micro-organism, whether viral, bacterial, fungal or other. As also mentioned above, several additional models of disease have varying levels of acceptance within medicine. Unlike germ theory all of these alternative perspectives operate on the assumption that most diseases do not have a single cause; instead they are seen as having multi-causal pathways. The most widely accepted of these are the immunity, genetic, environmental and – the focus of this book – lifestyle models of disease.

Like germ theory, understandings of immunity and genetics emphasise the role played in the development of disease by the body's own internal systems. Conceptions of immunity imply that bodies either win or lose the fight against disease from the inside (Martin 1994). A genetic understanding focuses on genetic mutations. These are argued to result in single gene disorders such as Huntington's chorea, in predisposition to diseases such as Alzheimer's and ovarian cancer, or more controversially, in behaviours deemed detrimental to health or disorders in themselves such as alcoholism, depression or obesity (Hubbard and Wald 1993; Wilkie 1994; Willis 1997a).

Both environmental and lifestyle theories of disease differ considerably from germ theory and theories of immunity and genetics because they utilise explanations for disease which emphasise the social rather than the biological. Environmental understandings emphasise factors external to the human body such as poor foodstuffs, environmental hormones, solar radiation, pollution, medicines, chemicals, substandard housing and sanitation, population density and the biological environment (Chavarria 1989; Hume-Hall 1990; Foster 1995). Environmental understandings can be seen as emphasising the social because environmental damage or contamination is frequently associated with industrial development, socio-economic inequality, working conditions and colonisation. Environmental illness is frequently politicised by activists who argue that various examples of disease (for example, the Love Canal and Woburn leukaemia clusters) result from the actions of governments or large companies (Gusfield 1981; Levine 1982; Brown and Mikkelsen 1990; Brown 1992).

Models of disease that focus on lifestyle behaviours are based on the assumption that certain diseases are somehow the result of an 'unhealthy lifestyle'. This understanding of disease emphasises the interrelationships between many variables in disease aetiology (Hughes 1994; Rutten 1995;

Cockerham 2000). However, unlike environmental models of disease which tend to posit individuals as victims of an unhealthy environment, lifestyle arguments emphasise the role of individual choice in health-related behaviours such as smoking, diet, exercise, alcohol, etc. 'Lifestyle theorists reject the notion, central to classic germ theory, that a single disease has a single aetiology. Instead they emphasise the interrelatedness of many variables in disease causality, principally those under the control of the individual' (Tesh 1990: 41)'. Thus lifestyle approaches stress personal responsibility for health. Furthermore, because lifestyle models provide an explanation for poor health where the factors considered to be determinants of disease are commonly perceived to be modifiable, a lifestyle approach is often orientated towards the future and emphasises the maintenance and fostering of health (Lawton 2002). It is this capacity to serve as an explanatory framework for health and disease prevention, not just for the causes of disease, which, in conjunction with an emphasis on the social, makes a lifestyle approach distinct from other explanatory models used in contemporary medicine.

Understanding disease and health in terms of lifestyle is not a new phenomenon in medicine. Relationships between the ways people live and the illnesses they develop have always been a focus for healers, western and non-western. Prior to the development of modern medicine it was common for physicians and healers to prescribe regimens of diet, activity, rest or penance as a way of treating disease (Black *et al.* 1984; Turner 1991a, 1996; Porter 1997). Cartwright describes Hippocrates as achieving success when treating his patients with the following regimen: 'a life of fresh air, controlled exercise, massage and hydrotherapy assisted by a liberal diet of suitable foods' (1977: 5). In seventeenth- and eighteenth-century Europe it was popular among physicians to advocate disciplined eating habits, exercise and sobriety (Turner 1991a). In non-western cultures, for example among the Hmong people, dietary and behavioural prescriptions are still invoked during life events such as pregnancy and childbirth (Julian and Easthope 1996).

Hughes (1994: 62) characterises such assumptions about relationships between ways of living and health as 'rules of life'. She suggests that such rules have been and continue to be:

> an essential aspect of every major medical or health belief system from ancient Egyptian, Chinese and Indian through to Greek and Islamic medicine and modern western medicine. They also perform important functions in non-literate medical systems such as those found in Aboriginal, Pacific and African societies.
>
> (Hughes 1994: 62)

Such rules of life are often based around widely held 'commonsense' ideas about disease and sickness, religious and moral beliefs, observation of disease and healing, and personal theories of the body and health held by practitioners of the various types of medicine and healing prevalent in each particular culture and historical epoch. Over the twentieth century there was a range of different ways in which medical people understood disease and health in terms of lifestyle. While many of these operated at the same time, for the sake of clarity they are described below in chronological order.

In the late nineteenth and early twentieth centuries, medical ideas about lifestyle and health were strongly informed by ascetic Christianity. A healthy lifestyle was perceived as one characterised by restraint, sexual abstinence and physical exercise. Various organised attempts to encourage this type of lifestyle include the Temperance Movement, the Boy Scouts and the Girl Guides. As such they were characterised by strong moral dimensions. Baden-Powell, the founder of the scouting movement, was on the Advisory Board of the International Anti-Cigarette League and asserted 'if every British boy will let cigarettes alone, we stand a good chance as a nation not only of holding our own, but of beating all competition' (cited in Welshman 1996: 1382). For Baden-Powell, smoking was a moral failing along with late rising, masturbation, drinking and betting. Active footballers were contrasted in Scouting for Boys with 'boys and young men, pale, narrow-chested, hunched-up, miserable specimens, smoking endless cigarettes, numbers of them betting' (cited in Welshman 1996: 1384).

Medical ideas about lifestyle from this period were also closely linked with nineteenth-century ideas about social problems associated with increasing urbanisation. A range of popular and academic theories arose at this time from philosophy and the developing fields of social science (political economy, sociology, psychology, geography), which attempted to explain social inequalities, social unrest and social patterns of mortality and morbidity. Such theories were frequently developed or interpreted in the light of inherent class and race bias to imply that poverty and sickness among the working classes, ethnic groupings and colonised peoples were the result of their style of living (Bulmer 1982).

Two different perspectives on this were taken. Public health reformers, sanitary engineers, some social theorists and governments with a collectivist ideology explained these differences in ways of living which induced patterns of disease and illness in terms of structural inequalities leading to a lack of nutritious food, poor living conditions and inadequate or outdated sanitary arrangements (Riley 1987; White 1994). The medical profession allied with various social interests and a political and economic climate which increasingly focused on the individual rather than the group adopted a lifestyle perspective which located the problem of differing ways of living in 'the individual rather than the organization of society' (White 1994: 208). Working-class or ethnic cultural lifestyles were by definition seen as unhealthy while white middle-class lifestyles were eulogised as being healthy (Woods 1978; Woodward and Woods 1984). For example, in a pamphlet written in 1878 a Dr Cambell based in South Australia identified poor and working-class mothers who weaned their babies during the summer months as the cause of high infant mortality rates:

> You may not have every comfort at your command that a rich man's baby has. It may be that your baby does not very regularly gets its daily bath, or is not waited upon with the attentive care that a special nurse would give it, or even does not sleep in the cosiest cot in the world. Deprived of all this it will survive but it will not survive if you depart entirely from the order of nature with its food [breastfeeding].
>
> (Cambell 1878)

By the mid-twentieth century when living standards had risen and the incidence of death from infectious disease had begun to fall, medical and lay understandings shifted away from issues such as nutrition and living conditions towards a vision where 'people were more apt to think of a healthy lifestyle in terms of the cleanliness of their own immediate environment, their own house and their bodies' (Martin 1994). While describing common perspectives on the body and disease in the mid-twentieth-century United States, Martin (1994) found that the major enemies to health were seen as germs attacking the surface of the body. Such threats could be controlled by minimising entry points for germs (such as wounds) and by removing germs through washing and disinfection before they could enter the body. In terms of understanding disease on the basis of lifestyle, this viewpoint clearly assigns responsibility for your own health, your family's health and the safety of those around you to your own habits and practices pertaining to cleanliness.

Cleanliness of the body understood in terms of killing germs initially emerged in the eighteenth century with the scientific discovery of microbes and continued to increase in prevalence throughout the twentieth century (Vigarello 1988):

> In the late eighteenth century with the scientific discovery of microbes, external signs of cleanliness were no longer considered sufficient. These theories were legitimised by science. Washing was seen to rid the body of microbes. Microbes were viewed as invisible monsters . . . all the more dangerous because of their tininess. . . . This notion of cleanliness has predominated in the twentieth century as medicine and science have become ever more revered.
>
> (Lupton 1994a: 34)

Fear of germs was a feature of lay and medical explanations for disease throughout the early twentieth century. This fear reached a peak in the 1950s (Lupton 1994a). Images from this time such as advertisements for Lysol disinfectant are easily recognisable. Patton describes the fear of germs at this time as verging 'on a mass psychosis. Germs are bad guys, foreign, unnegotiable, dangerous' (1986: 51). Martin (1994) provides the following quote from an elementary school textbook published in 1950:

> you must be on guard at all times. Disease germs are always on hand to attack. Be clean in everything you do. Remember, you must keep your hair and scalp, your fingernails and toenails, and your clothing clean as well as your skin. Keep fighting to destroy disease germs. Form habits that will protect you from harm.
>
> (Martin 1994: 26–7)

Despite this emphasis on personal responsibility for cleanliness, the connection between a healthy (clean) lifestyle and getting sick was still relatively fatalistic. Many diseases were not associated with germs (e.g. cancer) and health was seen as a passive status. In the quote cited above, germs are represented as active attackers to which the body has no natural defences. The common view of the body at this time was mechanistic. Bodies were machines which could wear out and break down. Some bodies seemed by their nature to be stronger than others (a strong constitution) but this is a passive strength because there is very little a person can do to increase or decrease resistance to disease (Martin 1994).

By the 1970s the mid-century understandings of a healthy lifestyle being a clean lifestyle and health being a passive status began to shift. There arose a different understanding about what constitutes a healthy lifestyle and about the relationship between this, individual responsibility and disease. The concept of health had changed from 'something that is viewed as the result of luck or biological inheritance to something that is achieved through personal volition. In other words, health has changed dramatically from being a passive to an active status' (White *et al.* 1995: 159). Notions of what constitutes a healthy lifestyle expanded considerably from mid-century notions about cleanliness to include a range of behaviours such as regular exercise, 'safe sex', not smoking, reducing alcohol consumption, using unleaded petrol, rejecting pharmaceutical drugs in favour of herbal or alternative medicines, eating organic foods and participating in screening tests for blood pressure and cholesterol (Goldstein 1992; Foster 1995; White *et al.* 1995). In addition, decisions about what constitutes a healthy lifestyle were increasingly based on the results of epidemiological research into the determinants of chronic diseases, public health policies and guidelines and popular and scientific theories of risk. This way of thinking has been termed the ideology of 'healthism' (Crawford 1978, 1980) or 'lifestylism' (Rodmell and Watts 1986). Lifestylism is characterised by a strong emphasis on individual responsibility for 'lifestyle choices'. 'Whether it is through exercise, diet, or stress management the avoidance of disease through personal effort has become a dominant cultural motif' (White *et al.* 1995: 160).

Influences on contemporary medical understandings of lifestyle

Reasons for the shift from health as a passive state to one that can be actively sought are complex (Nettleton 1995). As already discussed earlier, medical understandings of lifestyle and associated medical perceptions about the relationship between the way people live their lives and their states of health and illness are formed within a broad socio-historical context. The rest of this chapter addresses the relationship between the contemporary medical understandings of lifestyle outlined above and some of these wider socio-historical factors: those social processes associated with late/high modernity; demographic changes in western industrialised countries; local and international trends in government policy with regard to public health; a growth in the scope and influence of the fields of epidemiology and public health; and lay perceptions of lifestyle, health and disease.

Contemporary medical understandings of lifestyle, health and disease reflect and reproduce a range of social processes that characterise the advanced industrialised societies of the late twentieth century. The most important of these interrelated processes and changes in terms of their impact on medical understandings of lifestyle are the processes of rationality, ideologies of conservative individualism, the increasing commodification of health and health care and the 'risk society'.

The phrase 'processes of rationalisation' refers to the increasing rationalisation of social action claimed to be occurring in modern and late/high modern societies: 'Rational here refers to action which is calculable and impersonal' (Crook *et al.* 1992: 8). Rationalisation has a number of implications including the calculation of social action in terms of costs and benefits, an inflation of the importance of knowledge as a basis for action (such as positivist science), impersonality of power and authority, and the extension of control over natural and social objects (Brubaker 1984; Armstrong 1988; Crook *et al.* 1992).

A lifestyle approach which stresses individual responsibility for health through a cost/benefit analysis of behaviours and actions considered to be lifestyle choices and the prevention of disease in the future sits easily within the rationalist and calculative mood of late/high modernity. Such an approach represents a desire for control over the body (Featherstone *et al.* 1991; Synott 1993) and health understood in terms of rational choices and health care costs.

At the level of the organisation of health care this perspective leads on easily to economic rationalist approaches, and a preference for preventive programmes which emphasise the role of the individual rather than the state and which are motivated not by altruism but by a desire to reduce health care costs in the future:

The premise behind this type of thinking is that people get sick or injured and die prematurely not because of their lacking access to resources such as good housing, education and health care but due to self inflicted hazards like substance abuse, poor eating habits and violence.

(Remennick 1998: 27)

At the level of the individual, the rationality of late/high modernity contributes to a reconsideration of individual responsibility and individual identity. Under the conditions of late/high modernity the nature of individual experience is reconstituted. The individualist focus of modernity where 'one of the goals in life is to free oneself from social and cultural determination' (Gordon 1988a: 34) is highlighted as 'the individual increasingly stands alone, looking for security in the face of uncertainty and an implosion of knowledge-systems' (Annandale 1998: 19). Thus 'the body is the site of choices and options that individuals must make in a reflexive manner' (Giddens 1991: 8). 'As the visible aspect of the self the body is not passive but needs to be monitored by individuals as they balance opportunities and risks, virtually forced to design their own bodies' (Annandale 1998: 18). Under these conditions health is viewed as an individual responsibility and as a project to be worked on (Gordon 1988a; Bordo 1990; Giddens 1991). From this perspective health is a goal to be achieved as part of the ongoing project of enhancing the self. It is seen as a sign of 'competence, self control and self discipline' (Nettleton 1995: 50). This mode of thinking can be easily recognised in lifestylism.

The implications of this perspective are illustrated in the results of research that investigates the ways that people conceptualise health. Studies suggest that health is increasingly understood as an individual responsibility to be achieved through bodily maintenance and vigilance (Crawford 1984; Calnan 1987; Blaxter 1990, 1993, 1997). For example, Lupton (1995) reports the results of a study that interviewed white middle-class American men and women about their notions of health:

> health for both men and women was allied closely to physical standards that conformed to 'ideals' of being in 'shape'. Health was also something that could be achieved by deliberate intentional action involving the body such as dieting, having enough sleep and physical exercise.
>
> (Lupton 1995: 43)

Related closely with the 'self as project' is the commodification and commercialisation of bodies and health (Bordo 1990; Annandale 1998). As Turner (1996: 5) explains, 'Given the emphasis on selfhood in contemporary consumer culture the body is regarded as a changeable form of existence which can be shaped and which is malleable to individual needs and desires.' With the commodification of bodies, health becomes a commodity that individuals purchase, a possession (Gordon 1988a). Contemporary understandings of lifestyle are inextricably interlinked with the rise of consumer culture that is an inherent part of late/high modernity (Featherstone 1991; Nettleton 1995):

> health has become an essential prerequisite to participation in the youth valorising, sexualised, death-denying society in contrast to earlier times where modification of lifestyle was part of an ascetic or religious regime. Within this logic, fitness and slimness become associated not only with energy, drive and vitality, but worthiness as a person; likewise the body beautiful comes to be taken as a sign of providence and prescience in health matters.
>
> (Hughes 1994: 62)

The commodification of health has contributed to the popularity and development of lifestylism through an emphasis on the purchasing of health both in literal and symbolic terms through health care, health-related actions or health-related goods and services which are seen to represent a healthy lifestyle and thus 'health': for example, running shoes, exercise clothing, sports radios and sunglasses, exercise equipment or gym memberships (Glassner 1989). In addition, the commodification of health has contributed to consumerism within medicine and health care generally. While there is little consensus within sociology about consumerism and medicine, two issues which have relevance for contemporary medical and lay understandings of lifestyle and health are changes in the medical profession's monopoly over authoritative knowledge about health and illness and changing expectations about the role of medical care (Kleinman 1980).

Assertive patients who view themselves as consumers and see health and illness as a commodity to be purchased have become 'less willing to unquestioningly trust the [medical] profession's claims to expertise and ethicality' (Irvine 1999: 182). Other sources of health-related information are seen as worth considering and health-related advice becomes prevalent and profitable. This has contributed to the growth of alternative therapies and the self-help and fitness industries (Easthope 2004). Furthermore, along with a consumerist orientation, expectations about what medicine should actually offer patients (consumers) has increased. The provision of complementary therapies and preventive lifestyle advice is one aspect of the expanding medical package offered by doctors who are now competing with other service providers such as pharmacists, naturopaths and physiotherapists.

Associated with rationality, individualism and commodification is a fourth process associated with late/high modernity, that of the 'risk society': a situation where perceptions of risk are heightened and the identification and management of risks become a major concern (Beck 1990; Giddens 1991; Douglas 1992). Sociological arguments about a risk society emphasise that late/modern societies are characterised by a 'politics of anxiety' where the body is perceived as being under constant threat from external risks, for example the destruction of natural environments, chemical pollution and infections such as HIV/AIDS (Turner 1991b). This social climate, which emphasises risks and the making of informed choices on the basis of knowledge, is reflected in an approach to health that defines healthy or unhealthy lifestyles in terms of lifestyle risks (Beck 1990).

In late/high modernity where the body is 'reflexively mobilised' and issues of identity and health are made within a context of options and choices (Giddens 1991), risks to health become 'monitored by individuals as they balance opportunities and risks ... under conditions of considerable uncertainty' (Annandale 1998: 18). Understanding the determinants of health or disease in terms of lifestyle risks 'advocates a rationalistic, individualistic, prospective life perspective where maximising control and minimising uncertainty is seen as a superior goal' (Førde 1998: 1155).

In addition to the influence of various processes and assumptions associated with late/high modernity, medical ideas and practices are also constructed through a nexus of demographic change and government policies on public health. In the mid- to late twentieth century improved living conditions resulted in a decline in infectious diseases and an increase in chronic conditions with behavioural and social determinants (Hughes 1994). A growing elderly population in western countries was predicted, with resultant issues related to an over-burdened health service:

> The ageing of the population is a significant political and social issue for at least two major reasons. First the characteristics and prevalence of modern forms of degenerative disease are obviously closely related to the ageing of contemporary populations. . . . Secondly, the ageing of the population of industrialised societies has had a significant social impact on the economic performance of capitalism because of the dependent populations associated with ageing and retirement. Industrial societies will increasingly face a situation where significant proportions of their population are retired, elderly or disabled.
>
> (Turner 1996: 5)

In response to this demographic change those in charge of health policy turned their focus to disease prevention as it became apparent that increasing investments in technological medicine resulted in diminishing returns. Policies and health education campaigns based on a lifestyle approach to disease were widely implemented by governments in countries such as Australia, Canada and the United Kingdom (Palmer and Short 1994).

These policies made lifestyle issues such as nutrition, exercise, drug taking and sexual behaviours central to disease prevention (Duff 1999: 78), for example through the development of dietary guidelines (NHMRC 1992, 1997) and implementation of health promotion campaigns such as the QUIT campaign to encourage people to stop smoking. Such policies prioritise 'the self-seeking self-sustaining individual, the sovereign individual of liberal capitalism' (White 2000: 288). These policies were based on epidemiological research about lifestyle, disease and health and implemented through the public health system (Peterson and Lupton 1996; Australian Institute of Health and Welfare 1998). Epidemiology and public health are the two most significant 'legitimate' sources of information about lifestyle, disease and health. Thus contemporary medical understandings of lifestyle cannot be understood without closer examination of these fields.

Epidemiology and public health

Epidemiology has its basis in nineteenth-century efforts to systematically collate and analyse demographic information and to apply statistical methods to identify the distribution and determinants of epidemics of infectious disease (MacMahon and Pugh 1970; Susser 1973; Evans 1992; Pickstone 1992). As such, epidemiology clearly reflects the rationalist viewpoint through its reliance on the application of scientific methods of monitoring and measuring to the issue of population health (Petersen and Lupton 1996).

Epidemiology is the study of the distribution and the determinants of disease occurrence and outcome in humans. Epidemiological studies are usually observational and concentrated exclusively in humans. Epidemiology has always been one of the basic sciences in preventive and clinical medicine. Its first major impact was on the understanding of the aetiology and the natural history of infectious diseases and on the design and implementation of effective control measures for these diseases (Olsen and Trichopoulos 1992: v). With the reduction in infectious diseases in the twentieth century, increasing epidemiological attention was focused on identifying the determinants of chronic diseases associated with an ageing population and modern living conditions, such as osteoporosis, cataracts, stroke, diabetes, cancer, heart disease and arthritis. These diseases almost certainly have multiple determinants such as diet, genetic, psychosocial, and occupational factors and level of physical activity (and in some cases infectious factors):

> These multiple potential determinants may act alone or in combination. Also many of these diseases have long latent periods; they may sometimes result from cumulative exposure over many years and in other instances from a relatively short exposure occurring many years before diagnosis. For most of these diseases the relevant period of exposure is unknown. A third characteristic of these diseases is that they occur with a relatively low frequency despite a substantial cumulative lifetime risk. In addition, these conditions are not readily reversible.
>
> (Willett 1990: 4)

Epidemiologists generally work with a probabilistic conception of causality (e.g. Susser 1973; Rothman 1998). In addition, unlike germ theory (which presupposes that each disease has a single and distinct cause), epidemiology works with a web of causality approach (Krieger 1994). This is the idea that diseases are the result of complex interactions between a number of different factors. The following excerpt from an epidemiology textbook illustrates this approach to the causes of disease:

> One of the main aims of epidemiology is the study of the determinants of the occurrence of health-related events or conditions. Determinants may be biological, psycho-social, or health services related, and outcomes may be of qualitative or quantitative nature and refer to diseases, syndromes, symptoms, or functions, as well as natural history and evolution. Aetiological considerations are also fundamental to all stages of study design, analysis and interpretation. Therefore, teaching the concept of causation is an essential part of the teaching of epidemiology. Causation should be viewed in practice as probabilistic and should usually focus on categories or groups, rather than individuals.
> (Olsen and Trichopoulos 1992: 33)

Contemporary epidemiological conceptions of lifestyle are derived from this 'web of causality' approach and a focus on chronic diseases of civilisation considered to have social and behavioural determinants (Krieger 1994). The web of causality approach presumes that 'an individual's risk of contracting specific diseases depends on many interacting and interdependent variables' (Milner, S. 1998: 315). These include variables seen as individual risk factors such as lifestyle risks, inherited susceptibility and biological threat and those factors viewed as environmental or social risks. The web of causality approach 'depends, for its empirical survival on statistical techniques of multivariate analysis. The underlying model of pathogenesis assumes that improvements to the public's health depend on experts' ability to identify "risk factors" ' (Milner, S. 1998: 315). The key features of the epidemiological understanding of lifestyle are summarised below.

First, lifestyle is understood to refer to potentially modifiable social factors as contrasted with biological factors, which may or may not be modifiable (e.g. Twisk *et al.* 1997). Second, the conception of the social used in epidemiology understands social determinants of disease in terms of distinct behaviours or actions that can be isolated from other behaviours or actions for the purpose of research: for example, smoking or exercise rather than a general sense of a healthy or unhealthy lifestyle (e.g. Owen and Bauman 1992; Huang *et al.* 1996). The contemporary epidemiological approach views social factors such as socio-economic inequality, living conditions and employment as 'fundamental causes' of disease which are too distant and non-specific to be usefully investigated in medical research (Remennick 1998: 26; see also Pearce 1996). Instead, epidemiologists search for more proximate causes of disease such as lack of exercise, smoking, diet or occupational and environmental hazards (McKinlay 1993, 1994). This reductive approach to the social is closely related to the statistical methods used in modern epidemiology. Pearce argues that the statistical methods in vogue in late twentieth-century epidemiology (such as case control studies, logistic regression and exposure measurement) have contributed to an oversimplification in modern epidemiological thinking about social factors underlying patterns of health and disease, leading to a paradigm shift away from socio-economic and sociocultural studies to an almost exclusive focus on individualised risk. Earlier epidemiological perspectives that included structural factors such as social class and gender were replaced by 'a strong focus on statistical issues and paradigms. ... Most modern epidemiologists still do studies in populations but they do so in order to study decontextualised individual risk factors' (Pearce 1996: 679).

Risk in this context refers to the probability of getting a particular disease. Risk factors are those lifestyle behaviours or attributes which are deemed to increase the statistical probability of a certain percentage of an overall population who participate in these behaviours developing a particular disease (as are genetic environmental or physical attributes also associated with developing certain diseases). Behavioural risk factors that are considered to be modifiable by individuals are commonly termed lifestyle choices by epidemiologists. For example, the modifiable risk factors for coronary heart disease include low levels of physical exercise, drug taking including cigarette smoking and drinking alcohol, high levels of fat, sugar and salt in the diet, high blood cholesterol levels and stress (e.g. Willett 1990; Chang-Claude and Frentzel-Beyme 1993; Namekata *et al.* 1997; Rothman 1998). Other recognised risk factors for coronary heart disease that are not considered to be modifiable lifestyle factors include genetic predisposition and environmental factors including exposure to toxins and micro-organisms (Link and Phelan 1995).

It is important to recognise that despite epidemiological definitions that suggest risk can be easily quantified and understood, concepts of risk operate in many different ways in epidemiological understandings of lifestyle and disease. For example, lifestyle behaviours and attributes may be identified as 'risk factors' and be used to identify those 'at risk' from disease. In the case of sexually transmitted disease or cigarette smoking, people identified as participating in 'risky' lifestyle practices may also be defined as a 'risk' to others (Lupton 1994a: 137).

Next, in the epidemiological approach to lifestyle, the term lifestyle is generally only considered to refer to those behaviours or actions that can be shown to impact (usually negatively) on physical health. For example, while theoretically any of the behaviours and actions in which people regularly engage could be considered under the title of lifestyle, most are only considered by epidemiologists when they become associated with the development of physical disease. This is a reflection of a widespread biomedical understanding of health that is mechanistic and biological as distinct from other understandings of health that focus on perceptions of wellbeing or capacity to participate fully in social life. Risk as a topic and subject for epidemiological research has expanded rapidly since the 1960s (Heyman 1998). Skolbekken (1995), who in the 1990s conducted a search for the term risk in published epidemiological papers, found that risk factor research had become a dominant form of epidemiological research; also that this research was largely focused on non-iatrogenic risks such as lifestyle risk rather than risks associated with medications or treatments.

Finally, the epidemiological conception of lifestyle is focused on identifying lifestyle risks as the causes of disease. It is rarely focused on producing action or change among populations or by individuals (this is in contrast to the public health and health promotion version of a lifestyle approach discussed next). Epidemiology is primarily a research discipline interested in the 'why' aspects of disease and health; action on epidemiological research is carried out through public health/health promotion.

Epidemiology and public health have a long association (Holman 1992). The influence of epidemiological research into lifestyle risk factors on public health thinking became apparent in the early 1970s when it caused a shift from the classic late nineteenth-century focus on social institutions and mid-twentieth-century focus on social welfare to a micro-level focus on individuals, families and communities (Terris 1987). It should be noted that, as with the critique of risk factor epidemiology that came from within epidemiology, public health writers have also expressed concern about the increasingly individualistic focus of public health (Bunton and MacDonald 1992; Dean 1993; Pearce 1996).

Unlike in epidemiology, which has a coherent and consistent approach to lifestyle, a range of different and not necessarily compatible conceptions of lifestyle are found in contemporary public health. These different conceptions represent two distinct approaches. The first of these, seen by some authors as an early phase of the second approach (e.g. O'Connor and Parker 1995), is the epidemiologically driven, risk factor-focused health promotion that is sometimes also described as health education. The second is the new public health. These two different public health approaches imply quite different directions for the implementation of public health programmes/ interventions and offer quite different ways of understanding health and illness in terms of lifestyle.

Epidemiologically imbued risk factor health promotion is the most prominent public health discourse on lifestyle (Bruce 1991). This particular way of understanding the social causes of disease has been both popular and prominent because it is easily integrated into an individually focused health care system (Richmond 1997). Because risk factor health promotion utilises epidemiological data about the causes of disease, it shares a similar conception of lifestyle to the epidemiological discourse summarised above, i.e. lifestyle as behaviours and practices which are not considered in their social context but which instead are viewed as distinct and objective risk factors for various diseases (e.g. Russell and Buisson 1988; Badura and Kickbusch 1991; Pill 1991). Above all, behaviours and actions seen to be risk factors for disease are described as healthy (e.g. regular physical activity) or unhealthy (e.g. smoking) choices.

However, the lifestyle discourse found in risk factor health promotion is not identical to the epidemiological discourse of lifestyle. The first difference is related to conceptions and presentations of risk. The second is that public health is concerned with action aimed at preventing disease and improving health rather than understanding the causes of disease, or collecting general information about lifestyle factors in the population (as in epidemiology). Thus attention is focused on modifying lifestyles, as opposed to the epidemiological focus on lifestyle factors as a cause of disease. We are not arguing that public health is not a research discipline or that in practice this distinction is always apparent. Public health practitioners are frequently epidemiologists who do epidemiological research, and public health as a discipline has a significant research component. However, in relation to understandings of lifestyle, epidemiological texts do focus more closely on collecting information about lifestyle whereas public health texts concerned with risk factor health promotion focus more closely on controlling and modifying lifestyle behaviours and practices.

In relation to conceptions and representations of risk there are several differences between risk factor health promotion and epidemiology. The first is that in epidemiology risk is understood in terms of population risk. In contrast to this, in risk factor health promotion, lifestyle risks are frequently presented as the property of individuals. While public health practitioners sometimes work with population health, when addressing lifestyle risks their most common methods involve individually focused health education campaigns (Nettleton 1995; Richmond 1997).

Lifestyle factors commonly targeted in risk factor health promotion are smoking, exercise, nutrition, alcohol consumption, needle sharing during injecting drug use, some sexual practices and certain practices defined as lifestyle choices, e.g. exposure to the sun (Ross 1994; Krug 1995; Jonas *et al.* 2000; Stamfer *et al.* 2000). These behaviours are the target of lifestyle-focused health education in many countries including Canada, Australia, the United States and the United Kingdom. Fitzgerald (1994) makes the point that decisions about which behaviours are seen as lifestyle risks is not a direct reflection of the level of risk. He cites other behaviours that carry similar health risk such as mountain climbing or regular car driving that are considered acceptable, healthy and normal.

In lifestyle-orientated health promotion campaigns and health education, lifestyle risks are personalised and individualised (Kavanagh and Broom 1998). Risk factor health promotion subverts general epidemiological statements about population health risks into individually directed prescriptions for health. Rose (1992) describes this practice as a common irony in preventive medicine, because while widespread lifestyle changes will make a difference to community health they may make very little difference to the health of individuals:

> The prevention paradox: a preventive measure that brings large benefits to the community offers little to each participating individual. This distressing paradox implies that a response to honest health education is unlikely to be motivated powerfully by the prospect of better health. Whether or not a middle-aged smoker chooses to give up his cigarettes may affect his chances of being alive in twenty years time by less than ten percent. Similarly, a decision to lose some excess weight, to take regular exercise, or to use soft margarine in lieu of butter – each a prudent step to take – will make only a tiny difference to a particular person's health prospects.
>
> (Rose 1992: 12–13)

Another difference between the way that lifestyle is conceptualised in epidemiology and in risk factor health promotion is that in the former risks are understood in terms of levels of risk, in relation to other risks and in the context of general population health data, whereas in the latter lifestyle risks are frequently presented in all or nothing terms. As such, epidemiological research is being misrepresented. Bloor *et al.* use the word ethnostatistics to describe the process of interpreting statistical data in such a way as to make a convincing and legitimate-sounding argument (1991: 131). This process is common in public health applications of epidemiological data about lifestyle risks where the differences between various levels of risks are rarely mentioned because to do so would make it harder to argue for the adoption of various healthy practices or to attract funding for serious health issues (Petersen and Lupton 1996; Richmond 1997): 'Attempting to change behaviour involves enough problems without having to admit that everything we do carries a mix of costs and benefits. Professionals, therefore, will tend to present their advice in terms which avoid shades of grey' (Heyman 1998: 42).

Kavanagh and Broom (1998) demonstrate the impact of an overly simplistic use of risk in health promotion materials in their study of women who recorded an abnormal cervical smear result. These women had risk explained to them through public health information about cervical screening. They interpreted this information to mean that the risk of cervical cancer appeared and disappeared according to cervical smear results and treatment. That is, they considered there were two distinct states, at risk and not at risk. Their conceptions of risk are in contrast to an epidemiological conception of risk where all women are considered to be at some risk of developing cervical cancer, although their levels of risk might change according to circumstances.

A third difference between epidemiological understandings of lifestyle and those found in epidemiologically driven risk factor health promotion is that distinctions between risk and cause are blurred or non-existent in risk factor health promotion. In many health promotion texts, risk factors for the development of disease in populations are represented as the cause of disease in individuals. This is despite the widely accepted limitations of epidemiology to 'establish causal connections' (Heyman and Henriksen 1998: 41). Hughes (1994) argues that thinking about the relationship between lifestyle and health in a simplistic cause and effect way has several implications for contemporary conceptualisations of lifestyle and health. It changes health from being an ideal state to being a normative one. Ever expanding expectations about health have resulted in any state other than perfect health being perceived as a problem. In addition, perfect health, understood as being achieved through lifestyle modification, has become essential to full participation in society today. Next, if lifestyle is understood to be the cause of disease, then people afflicted with lifestyle diseases can be held accountable for their illness. Finally, current lifestyle-based explanations for disease stress prevention rather than treatment, so that 'the focus now is as often on "potential" illness as it is on real illness – on "virtual health" and "virtual disease" ' (Hughes 1994: 62; see also Kavanagh and Broom 1998).

Apart from differences in conceptions of risk, another major difference between epidemiological constructions of lifestyle and the constructions of lifestyle found in risk factor health promotion is that epidemiological texts reflect a focus on investigating lifestyle as a possible determinant of disease while, in contrast, risk factor health promotion texts generally take epidemiological knowledge about the relationship between lifestyle and disease as a given and focus on the modification and control of individuals' lifestyle behaviours and practices for the purpose of improving population health (Milner, S. 1998). This focus often involves empirical research orientated towards measuring the knowledge, attitudes and practices of given populations with the aim of developing programmes and interventions which will effectively result in the control and modification of lifestyle practices (e.g. Narayan and Venkat 1997). This type of lifestyle focus also involves the development and implementation of health education programmes which aim to educate individuals about lifestyle risks (Donahue and McGuire 1995; Duff 1999: 77):

> Such programs argue that people put their health at risk by smoking cigarettes, eating unhealthy food, drinking too much, and not exercising enough. In this discourse, the problem of illness is conceptualised in terms of individuals' non-compliance. Some people are said to have failed to give up full cream milk, for instance. Smokers are said to have 'failed to understand' that lung cancer and coronary heart disease are major risks of smoking.
>
> (Richmond 1997: 159)

Health education programmes have only limited success when assessed on the basis of measurable health outcomes (Beattie 1991; Mechanic 1994). Even when people do modify their behaviours, lifestyle changes are only maintained for short periods of time and are 'often limited to that segment of the population that is highly motivated to change, and the people who arguably really need to change are often impervious to health messages' (Richmond 1997: 159).

As a result of arguments that a risk factor health education lifestyle approach is flawed, public health policy makers at all levels have made statements about expanding the medical definition of lifestyle to take into account the socially embedded nature of lifestyle behaviours. This is evident in the World Health Organisation definition of lifestyle as 'patterns of behaviour choices made from alternatives that are available to people according to their socio-economic circumstances and to the ease with which they are able to choose certain ones over others' (Kickbusch 1986a: 118). Strongly associated with this shift in public health thinking is the approach termed the new public health that became popular in the mid-1980s (Ashton and Seymour 1988; Bruce 1991; Armstrong 1993).

The developers and supporters of the new public health claimed to have overcome the limitations of an overly simplistic risk factor lifestyle education approach to disease prevention. New public health policy replaces individual behavioural modification achieved through education about lifestyle in favour of enhancing people's life skills and environmental change where the environment is conceived as social, psychological and physical (McPherson 1992: 123). Ashton and Seymour define the new public health as an approach that:

> goes beyond an understanding of human biology and recognises the importance of those social aspects of health problems which are caused by lifestyles. In this way it seeks to avoid the trap of blaming the victim. Many contemporary health problems are therefore seen as social rather than solely individual problems; underlying them are concrete issues of local and national public policy; and what are needed to address these problems are 'Healthy Public Policies' – policies in many fields which support the promotion of health. In the New Public Health the environment is social and psychological as well as physical.
>
> (1988: 21)

The new public health was critiqued extensively throughout the 1990s by sociologists. We explore this in more detail in chapter 3. Here it is sufficient to note that some authors claimed that there is nothing very new about the new public health (e.g. Holman 1992) while others criticised the weaknesses in its paradigm (e.g. Petersen and Lupton 1996). Nevertheless it is widely acknowledged that the ideas and practices subsumed under the title new public health represent a quite different public health paradigm from the reductive epidemiologically driven public health (O'Connor and Parker 1995). In contrast to epidemiologically inspired risk factor health promotion the new public health has a much broader and more general conception of the social aspects of disease. In theory, the new public health operates with a biopsychosocial understanding of health which requires education and lifestyle modification to be part of general public policy, the workplace and education, not restricted to promotional campaigns (O'Connor and Parker 1995).

Unlike traditional public health which emphasised hygiene, mainstream medical thinking (germ theory) which emphasises the importance of medical care for health, or risk factor health promotion which focuses on a reductive collection of lifestyle practices considered to be risk factors for disease, the new public health viewpoint emphasises that lifestyle, socio-economic factors, the environment and health care systems all play an important role in the achievement and maintenance of health. The new public health claims to be directed not only to health issues in a narrow sense, but also to broader social, political and economic conditions that produce differences in health among different groups. For example, the five strategies for health promotion outlined in the Ottawa Charter framework are: building healthy public policy; creating supportive environments; developing personal skills; strengthening community action; and reorientating health services.

In this sense, then, the new public health conception of lifestyle is not one of socially isolated practices and behaviours. Instead, it aims to have a lifestyles understanding rather than a lifestyle understanding. The term lifestyle when utilised in new public health texts is not restricted to epidemiologically identified risk factors but is applied to a wider and more general conception of styles of living. Individuals' practices and behaviours are recognised as occurring within a context of structural and cultural factors. Rather than a focus on top-down education about lifestyle risks, the new public health emphasises community participation and empowerment. For example, Lupton (1999) describes how new public health discourses became evident in the curriculum for school physical activity programmes. These became framed in terms of self-esteem, holistic health, feeling good about oneself and being responsible.

Two features of this new public health approach to lifestyle, which make it very different from an epidemiological or a risk factor health promotion understanding of lifestyle, are the influences of sociology and wellness nursing. Sociological arguments about health have been integral to public health ideas about lifestyle since the late 1960s (e.g. World Health Organization 1985; Kickbusch 1986a, 1986b; Badura and Kickbusch 1991; Tannahill 1992; Waddell and Petersen 1994).

Sociology emphasises the role of social structures and inequalities on health, and requires a reflexive awareness of the cultural, historical and ideological basis of all public health thinking including ideas about lifestyle (e.g. Bunton and Macdonald 1992; Bunton *et al.* 1995; Flick 1998). From a sociological perspective, therefore, the epidemiological approach to lifestyle is reductive because it refers to a range of discrete behaviours and practices that can be isolated in risk factor studies. The health promotion perspective on lifestyle is also reductive when viewed from a sociological perspective because this conception of lifestyle carries connotations of easily made choices and 'styles' of life which might be easily abandoned for another 'style' of life if desired. This ignores the difficulties imposed by material constraints and the cultural and symbolic values of many of the behaviours dismissed so easily under the banner of lifestyle choices.

Wellness nursing expands available ideas about lifestyle to include the emotions and alternative/holistic understandings of diet and the environment (e.g. Schafer 1979; Pilch 1981; Keleher 1994; Storer *et al.* 1997). Wellness nursing originated in the 1970s and is strongly related to the primary health care movement, feminist nursing, alternative medicine and feminist and postmodern medical ethics and psychology (Petosa 1984; Chambers-Clark 1986). Textbooks about health promotion written for and by nurses reflect a strong interest in the emotional and psychosocial aspects of behaviours and behavioural change in a way that other public health texts do not (e.g. Faber and Rheinhardt 1982; Chin and Jacobs 1983). Wellness nursing also demonstrates an openness towards alternative/holistic therapies and these public health texts frequently advise that nurses apply a range of alternative/holistic healing modalities when attempting to modify or change a patient's lifestyle in order to improve health and prevent disease. For example, in her textbook *Wellness Nursing*, Chambers-Clark (1986) recommends that nurses teach their clients to make positive statements and use positive imagery to help them adopt and maintain healthy lifestyle practices such as taking up exercise or to give up unhealthy practices such as smoking. Note, however, that despite a rhetoric of empowerment, wellness nursing, like the new public health, continues the emphasis on control and modification of individuals' lives. Lay people are represented as patients (despite the use of the term client) who need help from nurses in the form of skill building, information and support in order to live healthier lifestyles.

In a study of the types of health promotion research being performed by the National Centre for Nursing Research (NCNR) in the USA, Pender *et al.* (1990) identified six categories of behaviour that were considered by researchers to comprise a health-promoting lifestyle. These were 'exercise, healthy nutrition, stress management, building supportive relationships, personal development, and taking personal responsibility for managing health through the appropriate use of health resources' (Lunney 1993: 250). A seventh category, 'concerning the reduction of risk behaviours such as smoking, alcohol use, and unsafe sex practices', did exist but was considered much less important (1993: 251). The majority of NCNR health promotion projects running in this period were concerned with the psychosocial aspects of healthy lifestyles, such as building supportive relationships and managing stress, rather than nutrition or exercise (Lunney 1993).

Lay understandings of lifestyle, health and disease

As discussed earlier in the chapter, lay and medical accounts of disease (including accounts of lifestyle) overlap and inform each other (Whittaker 1995). For this reason, and for purposes of comparison later in the book, the key features of lay perspectives on lifestyle in relation to health are outlined here.

The terms lay beliefs or lay understandings are often used to describe the 'commonsense,' 'folk' or non-scientific views about health and illness held by people who are not trained health professionals. However, as previously discussed in this chapter, the concept of layness in relation to understandings of health and illness is complex. It is unlikely that anyone living in contemporary western societies will hold views about health and illness that are uninfluenced by scientific medicine. Western societies are 'medicalised in a profound way' (Lupton 1997: 100). Lay people's general understandings will include elements taken from medical knowledge (Furnham 1988; Kerr *et al.* 1998; Popay *et al.* 1998). In circumstances where an individual or a relative has a medically diagnosed or managed illness they are even more likely to adopt medical explanations. For example, people with a chronic illness or caring for someone with such an illness often develop medical expertise surrounding that particular condition (Prior 2003; Hansen and Walters 2004). In 'actively searching for meaning patients and lay people can, and in most circumstances frequently do, adopt the expert/professionals' explanations and interpretations about their health and illness and come to accept such rationality' (Shaw 2002: 292).

Lay accounts of health that accumulate scientific and other data about the causes and distributions of illness in order to construct hypotheses about its causes and risks have been termed 'lay epidemiology' or 'popular epidemiology' (e.g. Davison *et al.* 1991, 1992; Brown 1992; Whittaker 1995). The term originated in an analysis of local discourses on health in South Wales where the authors found that lay people used their own aetiological frameworks and medical frameworks when talking about the causes of disease and disease prevention. The concept of lay epidemiology draws attention to areas of commonality between informal lay thinking and epidemiological reasoning about the causes of certain diseases. 'Lay and scientific "ologies" are not, of course, entirely congruent, but we discern a certain degree of overlap' (Davison *et al.* 1991: 7).

Furthermore, the concept of layness seems be based on a presumption that there is a clearly established medical viewpoint and lay viewpoint. However, lay people's views on health and disease differ according to a wide range of factors such as age, education, ethnicity, geographical location and health status (Bhopal 1986; Blaxter 1990; Howlett *et al.* 1992; Pierret 2003). Thus there are many different lay viewpoints and the differences among these may be as great as any differences between lay and medical knowledge. Furthermore, the views of different types of health professionals are not necessarily concordant or even scientific. Medicine includes a large number of different specialities and disciplines, many of which vary considerably in terms of preferred explanations for disease and the emphasis placed on scientific explanation. Thus the views about health and illness held by an epidemiologist might vary enormously from those of a nurse or a physiotherapist. In addition, health professionals 'belong to a wider culture', as do their loved ones (Heyman 1998: 21). They also have to explain health and illness in situations outside the context of their professional roles and may at times draw on non-medical models to do this (Hansen 2003a; Walters *et al.* 2005.

Nonetheless, despite the many instances of overlap between lay and medical understandings of disease they are still assumed to be very different (Shaw 2002). In studies of lay understandings 'it is noted that lay people often adhere to concepts of health, illness, disease and the body that may differ dramatically from the orthodox medical position' (Lupton 2002: 182). It is also a mistake to assume that lay people share understandings with health professionals even when they use the same terminology (Prior 2003).

The views of lay people about lifestyle and disease have been researched extensively (e.g. Blaxter and Paterson 1982; Blaxter 1990; Crossley 2002; Richards *et al.* 2003). Such research has produced complex and sometimes contradictory results about the ways that lay people use concepts of lifestyle when explaining health and illness. It is clear that lay people actively interpret medical explanations for disease in the light of experiences of illness, both their own and those of people they know. They have also been shown to resist explanations for disease which do not sit well with their wider beliefs, which imply that they are responsible for their ill-health or that they are likely to become ill or die prematurely (Blaxter 1983; Herzlich and Pierret 1987; Davison *et al.* 1991, 1992; Abrums 2000). Charles and Walters (1998) report this phenomenon in their study of age and gender in women's accounts of their health. They found that while the women interviewed frequently mentioned lifestyle and the need for healthy living, they attributed illness to a range of social, environmental and biophysical factors. The most common among these were ageing, financial situation and men. Other studies of lay perspectives on disease causation have found that lay people tend to emphasise biological factors, such as germs and genetic susceptibility, and factors such as stress and bad luck rather than lifestyle factors (Blaxter 1983; Calnan 1987; Richards *et al.* 2003).

It can be seen in the above example that lay people tend to neglect structural causes of health when explaining patterns of health and disease. This statement is supported by studies investigating lay people's views about social inequalities in health (Calnan 1987; Blaxter 1997; Popay *et al.* 2003). These studies show that people feel uncomfortable if it is suggested that states of health or disease are imposed by factors like poverty or the areas where they live. Thus, when asked to account for geographic or socio-economic patterns of health and illness, they tend to use lifestyle explanations that emphasise choices. Paradoxically, members of high socio-economic groups (who are at less risk of suffering from inequalities in health) show higher levels of awareness of social differences in the distribution of health and illness and are more aware of structural factors such as income, housing, the environment and access to opportunity than members of lower socio-economic groups (Calnan 1987; Popay *et al.* 2003). Thus 'those at risk of ill health may be less likely to acknowledge the social gradient of health' (Macintyre *et al.* 2005: 313).

It is clear that lay views follow 'particular patterns over time, tending to flow with the development and diffusion of related knowledge in the health sciences' (Angus *et al.* 2005: 2119). Recent studies suggest that lay people may be placing more emphasis on lifestyle as a factor leading to disease in response to exposure to many years of lifestyle-focused health promotion (Davison *et al.* 1992; Emslie *et al.* 2001). For example, Richards *et al.* found that respondents in their study 'consistently recognized the causative links between cardiac risk behaviours and heart disease' (2003: 712). After family history, the participants listed smoking, diet, being overweight and lack of exercise as causes. In this study the participants also described feeling responsible for heart disease either because this is how they already felt or because another person had told them they were 'to blame' (Richards *et al.* 2003: 713). Richards *et al.* (2003) also found that participants with a background of socio-economic disadvantage were more likely to feel guilty and to blame themselves for developing heart disease.

Diseases that have been the topic of lifestyle-focused health promotion campaigns, for example heart disease or lung cancer, are more likely to be described by lay people as being related to lifestyle (Calnan 1987; Zerwic *et al.* 1997; Mudge *et al.* 2005; Hansen 2003b). However, the majority of studies show the participants describing lifestyle factors such as diet, smoking or exercise as being only some of many possible causes (Richards *et al.* 2003; van Steenkiste *et al.* 2004; French *et al.* 2005). Lay explanations are often presented in complex aetiological narratives (Davison *et al.* 1991; Whittaker 1995) that rarely describe the cause of disease in terms of only one cause/risk. Thus lay people might attribute illness to any of a wide range of possible causes to which they give meaning by locating them within the wider context of a person's life. This process is clearly demonstrated by Gareth Williams in his (1984) study of people with rheumatoid arthritis. He found that asking people to tell him why they thought they had developed arthritis did not produce the list of causes he was expecting. Instead he found that each person made sense of their illness by locating it within their life story. Thus one participant discussed his arthritis in terms of his former occupation and difficult working conditions, another interpreted her illness in the context of her strong religious beliefs.

It seems that lay explanations also change depending on whether people are asked about disease in general, a specific disease or a disease that they (or someone close to them) have been diagnosed with (Popay *et al.* 2003). For example, French *et al.* (2005) conducted a study investigating the views of people who had recently had a myocardial infarct (MI) about the causes of heart disease. Their research participants described many different factors as causes of heart attacks in general, for example family history, stress, smoking. However, they often focused on 'just one of these factors as the sole necessary cause of their MI' (French *et al.* 2005: 1414). This was often described as an acute 'trigger'. The researchers also found 'there was often a great deal of reluctance for participants to blame their own behaviours for their MI' (French *et al.* 2005: 1415). Thus even when they described their heart attack as resulting from a lifestyle behaviour such as smoking or being overweight they were careful to explain this behaviour in a wider context such as being stressed, overworked or worrying about their family. Participants also spoke about the unpredictable nature of MIs.

There are many possible explanations for lay people's reluctance to explain disease as resulting from individual behaviours or actions. Some writers have suggested that people are understandably reluctant to attribute personal responsibility for illness as this type of explanation leads to negative consequences such as feelings of guilt (Davison *et al.* 1999). Others have argued that it may be related to 'a clear distinction within lay logic between health and disease' where health and disease are not seen as opposites (Williams 1983; Calnan 1987). From this perspective it is possible to be strong, fit and healthy and have a disease (Nettleton 1995). 'Ideas about the causation of disease are therefore not the same as ideas about the maintenance of health' (Nettleton 1995: 45). This argument is supported in a large number of studies of lay perspectives on health that suggest there 'appears to be a powerful moral imperative associated with health and the normality of health' (Popay *et al.* 2003: 3). Popay *et al.* (2003) suggest that many of the studies where lay people explain health and illness in terms of lifestyle are in fact asking questions about health rather than disease. Arcury *et al.* (2001) and Eyles *et al.* (2001) investigated lay understandings about the determinants of health and meaning of health maintenance behaviours. Both of these studies found that lay people in the USA and Canada gave biopsychosocial explanations for health. Personal health practices such as diet, drinking water and exercise were described by participants as being the most important. However, these were closely followed by a range of factors, such as social contacts, health care, education, employment and staying busy.

Davison *et al.* (1991) suggest that another reason for lay people's disinclination to accept the arguments about lifestyle and disease which they encounter in health promotion and epidemiology is the seemingly contradictory evidence they see for themselves: friends who have smoked and have not developed lung cancer; people with lifestyles characterised by lack of exercise and diets high in fats who do not develop coronary heart disease (Whittaker 1995; Emslie *et al.* 2001). Lay risk models are quite different to the 'mathematical risk models used by doctors' (Misselbrook and Armstrong 2002: 1).

Lay people in the late twentieth and early twenty-first centuries are part of a risk society where risk consciousness is heightened and people experience a 'widespread but diffuse sense of insecurity which is channelled into concerns about individual health' (Heyman 1998: 19). Studies show that lay people show an increased concern about lifestyle and health and seem increasingly to feel that the 'modern Western diet and lifestyle are uniquely unhealthy and are the main causes of contemporary epidemics of cancer, heart disease and strokes' (Fitzpatrick 2001: 1). For example, Barskey (1988) and Barskey and Borus (1995) using survey data demonstrate that despite improvements in health over the previous thirty years, Americans describe themselves as feeling dissatisfied with their health and concerned about the impact of their lifestyle on their health.

Unlike epidemiological concepts of risk which are abstract, population based and mathematical, lay ideas about lifestyle and risk are tied into each individual's own explanatory models and the folk and commonsense knowledges of their family and community (Douglas 1992; Green 1997). This results in quite different conceptions of risk from those used in epidemiology and may mean that lay people make their own, different interpretation of risk information conveyed by health professionals and health promotion campaigns. First, lay understandings of lifestyle risk are personalised. In lay accounts risk is described as 'the property of an individual, an embodied sign of future disease, and risk factors are reified properties which an individual has or does not have' (Whittaker 1995: 9). Thus lay people often describe a polarised understanding where risk is seen as being either high or low/non-existent (Davison *et al.* 1991; Kavanagh and Broom 1998). This polarised understanding of risk is in contrast to the epidemiological understanding, where populations are the units of analysis and statements about risk cannot be translated into a simple calculation of 'any individual person's likelihood of contracting any particular disease' (Whittaker 1995: 9). Furthermore, in the epidemiological conception, risk is seen as graduated. Thus any member of a population has some degree of risk.

Next, in lay accounts the term risk is often used to refer to danger and to bad luck interchangeably. Thus for lay people health risks are not the readily quantified result of risk calculations; instead they are unpredictable dangers (Douglas 1992; Emslie *et al.* 2001; Misselbrook and Armstrong 2002). Consequently, lay people recognise that attempts to predict health risks are fallible. For example, studies investigating lay views on health risks for heart attack have frequently found that even when research participants offer complex models for identifying people at greater risk of heart disease and profess the 'opinion that heart disease is to some extent preventable or postponable, the idea that it could happen to anyone (at any time) is omnipresent' (Davison *et al.* 1991: 14).

Like to the conflation of risk with bad luck or danger, lay accounts also conflate risk and cause. Thus epidemiological studies describing risk factors for diseases such as heart disease, cancer or diabetes are often interpreted causally by lay people (Davison *et al.* 1991; Nettleton 1992). Heart attack patients, for example, often included cardiovascular risk factors among their lists of the possible causes of their heart attack (Davison *et al.* 1991; Angus *et al.* 2005; French *et al.* 2005). Thus lay understandings of lifestyle, as described in a number of sociological studies, are characterised by features that at times make them quite different from the formalised and medically legitimate understandings of lifestyle found in epidemiology or public health (Pierret 1993; Salonstall 1993; Whittaker 1995; Popay *et al.* 1998).

However, it remains unclear how individual doctors construct lifestyle as an explanatory concept and how their understandings and different types of doctors' understandings of lifestyle relate to each other and to those of lay people. Several studies of GPs' and family doctors' views on lifestyle, health and disease suggest that they may hold views similar to lay people (Williams and Boulton 1988; Eyles *et al.* 2001). These studies will be reviewed in detail in the following chapter.

Conclusion

This chapter began with a discussion of explanatory frameworks within medicine that argued that at any one time, several different explanatory frameworks are operating within medicine and thus being used by doctors to make sense of health and illness. These frameworks vary for a number of reasons. They are based on different medically accepted, scientific models of disease, for example genetic and environmental models. Furthermore, medical explanatory frameworks are not an objective representation of the natural world; rather, like\other scientific knowledges, they are socially produced and thus imbued with the values and beliefs of their originating culture and time period (Gordon 1988a). Adding complexity to doctors' understandings of disease and health is the issue of medical practice. Doctors interpret formalised medical explanatory models within the context of their clinical and life experiences (Siegler 1981). Medical knowledge is also constructed through interaction between doctors, between other medical people and between doctors and their patients (Helman 1985a; Atkinson 1995). Thus doctors make sense of health and disease in a complex fashion that transcends the traditional sociological characterisations of medical knowledge (i.e. the medical model, the disease/illness distinction and the medical/lay dichotomy).

Lifestyle-focused explanatory models are of great interest to sociologists because they are social models of disease. Contemporary medical understandings of lifestyle appear to be markedly different from other medical explanatory frameworks currently in vogue. This is because a lifestyle approach assumes a multi-causal aetiology, addresses the social determinants of disease and provides an explanatory framework for health and not just biological disorder (disease). While lifestyle models of disease are a long-standing feature of medical thought, contemporary medical understandings of lifestyle are different from earlier ones because they reflect the cultural, demographic and structural situation of late advanced capitalist societies. Contemporary lifestyle-focused explanatory frameworks are characterised by an emphasis on individual responsibility for health and rely on the calculation and management of risks.

Contemporary medical understandings of lifestyle reflect and reproduce wider social understandings of lifestyle, bodies and health (Fitzgerald 1994; Hughes 1994; Bunton and Burrows 1995). To demonstrate this, contemporary medical and lay understandings of lifestyle were located within their social and cultural context. This context included: epidemiology, public health and preventive health paradigms; the ideology of 'healthism/ lifestylism' and associated shifts in conceptions of health (Crawford 1978, 1980; Rodmell and Watts 1986; White *et al.* 1995); social processes associated with late/high modernity such as rationality, ideologies of individualism, the increasing commodification of bodies, health and health care and the 'risk society' (Beck 1990; Giddens 1991; Turner 1996; Willis 1997b; Annandale 1998); also the nexus between demographic changes associated with ageing western populations and government policies on public health.

In addition, while medical understandings of lifestyle include a range of sociocultural values within their nosology the ways that formal medical knowledges use lifestyle to make sense of health and illness differ significantly from those of epidemiology and public health and also from the ways that lay people have been shown to understand lifestyle (Blaxter 1990, 1997; Davison *et al.* 1991, 1992; Pierret 1993; Whittaker 1995). Comparisons are frequently made between the variable and socially embedded nature of lay understandings of lifestyle and the reductive and universalistic nature of epidemiological understandings (Nettleton 1995; Skolbekken 1995).

Medical understandings of lifestyle also differ from sociological understandings of lifestyle, health and illness. Speaking broadly, sociological conceptions of lifestyle are closely linked with an awareness of life chances and structural/cultural factors that interact with individual lifestyles. In contrast, medical understandings of lifestyle are largely derived from epidemiological studies of behavioural risk factors for disease. They tend to be individualist and linked closely with programmes designed to prevent disease by modifying people's lifestyles. Thus while a sociologist might argue that the fundamental causes of disease lie in answers to questions such as 'Why do these people work in dangerous jobs?', 'Why do these people live in houses exposed to environmental toxins?' or 'Why are increasing numbers of young women starting to smoke cigarettes?', the epidemiologist would argue that 'workplace exposure to asbestos causes cancer and lung disease', 'the childhood leukaemia cluster in Cumbria is caused by radiation exposure from nearby nuclear power plants' and 'increasing numbers of lung cancer cases in women are the result of more women smoking cigarettes' (Link and Phelan 1995; Remennick 1998).

In the next chapter we begin our discussion of the sociological critique of medical understandings and applications of the lifestyle model by exploring the differences between sociological and epidemiological conceptions of lifestyle in more detail. We present the major sociological criticisms of the more common epidemiological conceptions of lifestyle and draw on evidence from epidemiology and public health to discuss the limitations of contemporary medical understandings of lifestyle as used in disease prevention and health promotion programmes.

2   Sociological and medical conceptions of lifestyle

Introduction

Le Fanu describes medicine as being 'seduced by social theory' in the second half of the twentieth century (1999: 312). Arguments about the role of social factors (lifestyle) in the aetiology of common diseases and an associated shift in focus from acute care to disease prevention were adopted with considerable enthusiasm by a range of medical researchers, doctors, policy makers, groups such as the World Health Organization and governments who viewed these new ideas as a possible solution to expensive hospital-orientated medical services (Puska 1985; Russell and Buisson 1988; Ornish et al. 1990; Badura and Kickbusch 1991; Pill 1991; Dines and Cribb 1993). Sociologists also viewed medical adoption of a social framework for disease with considerable favour. Epidemiological research into the behavioural and social basis of many diseases was seen to provide medically accepted scientific evidence to support longstanding sociological arguments that diseases are best understood as being socially produced and distributed, shaped by factors such as gender, ethnicity, employment patterns and socioeconomic inequalities (White 2002).

A lifestyle approach to health and disease prevention was also greeted with widespread optimism within medicine and by other disciplines as an indication that the limitations of a medical system focused on acute care were being recognised and that a new biopsychosocial approach to health and disease was being developed. This would overcome the doctor-focused perspective of the mainstream medical approach to disease, empower individuals and have greater potential in reducing inequalities in morbidity and mortality (Engel 1981; Monaem 1989).

However, it became clear to many sociologists that medical understandings of lifestyle and the social 'causes' of disease and poor health were very different from those used in sociology. Furthermore, evidence accumulated that the individualised conceptions of the social used in medical fields such as epidemiology were not resulting in successful disease prevention programmes. A sociological critique of medical understandings of lifestyle came into being. This critique was in two parts. The first was concerned with assessing the usefulness of medical ideas about lifestyle as a framework for disease prevention. This critique forms the basis of this chapter which also establishes the core differences between mainstream sociological understandings about the social determinants of disease and those used in epidemiology, public health and health promotion. The chapter draws extensively on studies from within epidemiology and public health in support of sociological claims that attempts to change individual lifestyles will achieve very little in terms of preventing disease or creating healthier societies. The second cultural aspect of the sociological critique of medical understandings of lifestyle is presented in chapter 3.

Does epidemiological research focused on lifestyle provide an effective explanation for patterns of health and illness?

As stated in the previous chapter, 'epidemiology is the paramount supplier of facts, premises and "bases of action" for preventive medicine and health promotion' (Førde 1998: 1155). The epidemiological approach to lifestyle derives from a multicausal model of disease that includes social and environmental factors and it is primarily concerned with identifying risk factors for disease (Skolbekken 1995; Pearce 1996). These are identified through the collection of population health and demographic data and statistical analysis.

However, the focus of epidemiological research is prediction rather than understanding (Peretti-Watel 2004). Thus the 'internal mechanisms of the multi-factorial model – the relative weight and relevance of risk factors and how they operate to produce specific disease – are quite vague and underspecified' (Shim 2002: 137). Sociologists and some medical anthropologists (as well as critics within epidemiology and public health) have queried the basis of many of the epidemiological claims about lifestyle and disease, and argued that epidemiological understandings of lifestyle are not effective ways of explaining patterns of health and illness.

Epidemiological explanations have been criticised for representing disease and lifestyle in a universalistic fashion that masks the value-driven nature of scientific research. Decisions about what diseases to investigate, how the investigations should be designed, the interpretation of results and the translation of these into interventions reflect particular social and cultural contexts. This is rarely acknowledged within epidemiology or by those disciplines that make use of epidemiological data (Lock and Gordon 1988a, 1988b; Shim 2002). For example, Potts (2004) argues that the epidemiological focus on individualistic and biological risk has made it difficult for environmental explanations for breast cancer to be investigated. Similarly, studies of lifestyle risks rarely investigate behaviours or practices often perceived as healthy, for example playing competitive sport or undergoing medical treatment (Skolbekken 1995).

Shim argues that 'epidemiological work on disease incidence and causation have always been sites where racial, class and gender orderings are visible and constitutive' (2002: 130). For example, epidemiological research investigating HIV led to risk categories for infection that were almost impossible to shake off even when they were revealed as inaccurate or less than useful. These demonstrated stereotypical understandings about sexuality, race and drug use. According to Shim (2002) the multifactorial model used in epidemiology explicitly acknowledges the role of social factors such as race or gender in epidemiological studies. However, these are rarely viewed as socially constructed categories; rather, they are seen as naturally occurring. In addition, 'because epidemiological findings emerge from research in which the unit of analysis is the individual, processes and dynamics of disease risk and causation are systematically reduced to that level' (2002: 132). Thus the complex relationships between a wide range of factors is reduced to a focus on 'the independent characteristics and behavioural choices of decontextualised persons' (2002: 133). (Similar arguments have been raised by Le Fanu 1986; Kaplan 1988; Germov and Williams 1999; Skolbekken 1995.)

Some epidemiological research fails to encompass the variations which occur within populations because it has relied too heavily on specific lifestyle behaviours which have been statistically associated with morbidity or mortality in population health data (Dean *et al.* 1995; Popay *et al.* 1998; Kowal and Paradies 2005). Global statistical correlations hide ethnic and gender variations. For example, Asian immigrants to Britain have high coronary heart disease rates despite having lower cholesterol, lower blood pressure readings and lower rates of tobacco consumption than non-immigrant Britons (Mckeigue and Marmot 1988). Similarly, women (unlike men) with high blood cholesterol are not statistically associated with higher mortality rates from cardiovascular disease in particular or with mortality in general (Hulley *et al.* 1992; Jacobs *et al.* 1992).

Epidemiological research into lifestyle, it is argued, also reflects the white/male-centred bias of medical research in general. Epidemiological research into lifestyle and disease is generally focused on adults and, more often than not, on white adult men rather than adult women or people from different racial or ethnic backgrounds (Saggers and Grey 1991; Foster 1995). The epidemiological focus on white men is also a reflection of the connection between lifestyle research and the diseases of middle-aged men. Although men and women are both affected by lifestyle diseases such as cardiovascular disease, lung cancer and adult onset diabetes, popular and medical constructions have often represented them as diseases which are a major problem for middle-aged men (e.g. Waldron 1983; Verbrugge 1985; Sabo and Gordon 1995).

At its basis, sociological concern about epidemiological attempts to address social determinants of health by focusing on lifestyle reflects a fundamental difference between sociological and epidemiological understandings of lifestyle and health (Phelan *et al.* 2004). Mainstream sociological perspectives on causes of disease emphasise the socially embedded nature of the behaviours and attributes considered in an epidemiological approach to be lifestyle risks. For example, both the following sociological definitions of lifestyle give emphasis to structural and cultural factors associated with behaviours and actions related to health. Cockerham (1995: 90) defines health lifestyles as 'patterns of voluntary behaviour based on choices from options that are available according to their [individuals'] life situations'. Abel describes health lifestyles as 'patterns of health related behaviour, values and attitudes adapted by groups of individuals in response to their social, cultural and economic situation' (1991: 900). Thus, from this sociological perspective, lifestyle factors and lifestyles are constrained by material resources in addition to cultural and symbolic values. Sociological arguments about social location and health focus on how life chances shaped by an individual's social location impact on their health, for example through social opportunities, material advantage/disadvantage, living conditions, working conditions and access to education and social support:

> Individual lifestyle choices are socially shaped, and [a] focus on them as an explanation of the cause of disease misses the social factors involved in the production of individual actions . . . there are a range of mediating social factors that intervene between the biology of disease, individual lifestyle, and the social experience shaping and producing disease.
>
> (White 2002: 2)

In many epidemiological studies about the causes of common diseases such as heart disease, class is excluded from the statistical analysis because it (inequality and socio-economic status) has the largest causative impact on patterns of disease (White 2002: 64; Terris 1996: 434). By reducing the complex causes of disease to individual risks, contemporary epidemiology 'systematically obscures the social forces that produce and reproduce the poverty and inequality which give rise to disease' (White 2002: 64). White argues that over-reliance on statistical risk factor research designs in positivist epidemiology has meant that epidemiologists are engaged in producing vast amounts of largely unrelated data that do not help to explain patterns of disease (2002: 64).

> When epidemiologists focus on the proximate causes of disease, diet, cholesterol and hypertension for example, they individualise the causes of disease and miss the distal social causes. As Link and Phelan (1995) argue, we need to contextualise risk factors so as to see how individuals are exposed to them and have limited access to resources to respond to them. It is the lack of resources to respond to risks that is the fundamental cause of disease patterns. If we want to change the

patterns of disease then we must change the distal, not the proximate causes.

(White 2002: 62)

The sociological position on lifestyle is frequently attributed to Weber (1978) who considered that while choice is 'the major factor in the operationalization of a lifestyle', 'the actualization of choices is influenced by life chances' (Cockerham *et al.* 1997: 325). Life chances are the chances that people have because of their position in life. This includes factors such as gender, age, education, employment, income and property as well as rights, norms and social relationships. 'Hence, lifestyles are not random behaviours unrelated to structure but are typically deliberate choices influenced by life chances' (Cockerham *et al.* 1997: 325).

In addition, when discussing the social, cultural and economic situation within which patterns of health are formed, sociological writers have emphasised that the social causes of ill-health are closely related to social inequalities (Navarro 1976, 1986; Epstein 1978, 1990; McKee 1988). In fact, inequality is viewed by many sociologists as *the* most important social factor impacting on health and disease (Wilkinson 2005, 1996). 'The outcome of the unequal distribution of political, economic and social resources necessary for a healthy life is the social gradient of health' (White 2002: 1). As evidence, sociologists point to the differential health outcomes of different social groups such as men and women, indigenous and non-indigenous Australians, rural/urban dwellers, the unemployed and students (Davis and George 1990; Saggers and Grey 1991; Germov 2004).

These writers argue that the individualist focus of epidemiological research reflects a failure of the state to acknowledge or take responsibility for situations within which health-related behaviour choices are made, for example the constraints imposed by unhealthy working conditions or the regulation and advertising of commodities such as tobacco or alcohol (Terris 1998). The medical profession has also been criticised for promulgating the commodification of health care and producing/reproducing a perspective where the causes of ill-health are physically located within an individual, thus masking the diffuse and complex relationships between social factors such as socio-economic inequality and poor health (McKee 1988; Pearce 1996). Sociologists draw extensively on research that demonstrates a strong association between socio-economic status, inequality and mortality (Link and Phelan 1995; Heslop *et al.* 2001; Phelan *et al.* 2004; Iribarren *et al.* 2005; Wilkinson 2005).

The type of lifestyle approach advocated by social scientists is also a reflexive and critical one that situates contemporary ideas about lifestyle, health and disease within a wider ideological and socio-historical framework (e.g. Bunton and Macdonald 1992; Dines and Cribb 1993). The theoretical perspectives that have resulted in a reflexive stance within sociology include Foucauldian writings and works by other writers using a

Foucauldian perspective (e.g. Armstrong 1982, 1983, 1995; Nettleton 1992), postmodernism (e.g. Fox 1992, 1993, 1999), medical anthropology (e.g. Lock 1985, 1986; Gordon 1988a; Martin 1990) and feminist writing (e.g. Ehrenreich and English 1974; Harding 1991; Bransen 1992). None of these perspectives which advocate a critical self-awareness by researchers and policy makers have been influential in the fields of epidemiology or applied public health to any extent. Thus it is unusual for proponents of either medical field to consider their own arguments about lifestyle and disease as only some of many possible ways to approach such issues.

There are important exceptions to reductive asocial epidemiology. For example, a number of epidemiologists explicitly practise a 'social epidemiology' that addresses the wider social context of individual risks and lifestyles (Marmot *et al.* 1978, 1991; Karasek and Theorell 1990; Syme 1996; Davey Smith 1996; Davey Smith *et al.* 1997; Wilkinson 2004, 2000a, 2000b). Social epidemiology uses epidemiological methods of statistical analysis to explore the relationship between inequality, income, gender, location, occupation, etc. and morbidity and mortality. Unlike mainstream epidemiologists, social epidemiologists work with concepts very similar to those used in sociology, geography and anthropology. While there is debate among social epidemiologists about the relative impact on morbidity, health and mortality of material conditions, income inequality, social status and psychosocial factors such as stress and anxiety, there is a widespread consensus that individual behaviours and risk factors cannot be understood outside their social context and that this includes historical, cultural, political and economic processes.

George Davey Smith and colleagues such as John Lynch use epidemiological methods to investigate the relationship between material conditions and health in an attempt to better understand socially distributed patterns of health and disease (Davey Smith *et al.* 1997; Lynch *et al.* 2004). Instead of a narrow risk factor approach to lifestyle, this neo-materialist approach focuses on structural issues and material conditions such as housing, employment and social infrastructure to demonstrate links between, for example, poor housing conditions and mortality (Dedman *et al.* 2001). The neo-materialist interpretation is 'an explicit recognition that the political and economic processes that generate income inequality influence individual resources and also have an impact on public resources such as schooling, health, care, social welfare, and working conditions' (Lynch *et al.* 2000: 1203).

The Whitehall 1 and 2 studies used epidemiological methods to investigate gradients of mortality among civil servants (Marmot *et al.* 1978, 1991). These studies have paid closer attention to variations within and across populations and the social contexts of individual risks and were 'important in drawing attention to the possibility that excess mortality is not just a matter of the cumulative effect of conventional risk factors' (Popay *et al.* 1998: 623):

Even more importantly what these studies established was the limited impact of lifestyle factors on health variations. Marmot and his co-workers controlled for diet, smoking, exercise and blood pressure in their sample and found that these factors could explain only one-third of the variance in disease between grades.

(White 2002: 73)

Richard Wilkinson is a social epidemiologist who has focused much of his research on investigating causal relationships between inequality and health (1996, 2000a, 2002b, 2005). A key feature in his work is a focus on the role played by the meaning of material factors in the causal relationship between inequality and disease. Wilkinson argues that lower social status (relative poverty, social exclusion) is associated with chronic stress and social exclusion (a lack of social support) that has a physiological effect. Wilkinson views stress as socially induced, the result of social conditions rather than an aspect of an individual's psychological makeup.

His psychosocial argument provides an explanation for why the richest countries are not necessarily the healthiest and why improvements in technology and wealth, in countries like the United States, have not led to commensurate improvements in health (Marmot and Wilkinson 1999). According to Wilkinson's argument, attempts to improve health by modifying individual lifestyles (even when this is achieved by improving income, education or social position relative to others) will not result in reductions in disease across populations unless these lifestyle changes are accompanied by an overall reduction in social inequality and thus an increase in social cohesion (Wilkinson 2000a: 582). This argument provides an alternative to the standard epidemiological lifestyle accounts focused on health behaviours and it has also been described as an alternative to materialist explanations such as Marxist accounts and neo-materialist interpretations such as those of George Davey Smith.

However, Wilkinson's arguments have been criticised for overemphasising the relative importance of perceptions of inequality and downplaying the structural causes of inequality and material factors (Lynch *et al.* 2000; Mutaner and Lynch 1999). Critics such as Mutaner and Lynch (1999) argue that Wilkinson's psychosocial explanation does not pay sufficient attention to how income inequalities are generated in the first place. 'The model ignores class relations, an approach that might help explain how income inequalities are generated and account for both relative and absolute deprivation' (Mutaner and Lynch 1999: 59). They (and others) also suggest that the favourable health measures seen in wealthy countries with greater income equality may in fact be a reflection of 'greater general social equality' that, in addition to reducing differences between incomes, has also resulted in widespread access to quality education, health care, suitable housing and social welfare (Lynch and Davey Smith 2002: 550). Recent reviews of research into the relationships between income inequality and health also suggest that in countries (other than the United States) where basic material needs are met, the relationship between income inequality and health is not as straightforward as Wilkinson states (Lynch *et al.* 2000; Lynch and Davey Smith 2002). Wilkinson's argument that health inequalities can be improved by alleviating social stress through a focus on social cohesion has also been criticised as a basis for social policy. Coburn argues that this way of explaining health inequality is open to abuse by governments who may view it as providing an excuse to neglect structural and material measures while focusing instead on building social capital through neighbourhood and community groups (Coburn 2000, 2004; Wilkinson 2000b).

Social epidemiology is a vibrant multidisciplinary field, as is evidenced by the frequent publications by social epidemiologists in sociological, epidemiological and mainstream medical journals. Social epidemiologists continue to trial new methods of investigating the interconnections between social dimensions such as education, occupation, income, housing, ethnicity, gender and age and health. They also make use of multidimensional conceptions of health and draw on qualitative research to enrich their statistical analyses. However, despite the apparent explanatory power of social epidemiology, simpler lifestyle/risk factor epidemiology continues to be the more commonly used source of epidemiological knowledge about lifestyle in medical fields and provides the legitimation for many health promotion programmes. In the next section we examine how successful such programmes have been in preventing disease.

Do health promotion programmes aimed at modifying lifestyle risk factors produce improvements in health and prevent disease?

Despite considerable amounts of research aimed at providing support for claims that health and disease can be explained in terms of lifestyle and that certain diseases could be prevented by lifestyle modifications, the impact of lifestyle on mortality and the development of various diseases remains obscure. A generally healthy lifestyle does seem to result in improved levels of health and wellbeing. For example, members of the Seventh Day Adventist Church, who take regular exercise, eat a vegetarian diet and neither smoke nor drink, have lower rates of certain diseases than the general population. However, the health outcomes of lifestyle changes at the level of isolated behaviours and practices are contested from many different sites, including from within the medical profession. See, for example, the following quote from David Weatherall, Director of the Institute of Molecular Medicine at Oxford.

While clinical trials have shown the benefits of stopping cigarette smoking, many of the changes in lifestyle that are being promoted by Western governments are based on information lacking in solid evidence.

It is unpardonable to try and alter the diet of an entire population without sufficient information.

(Weatherall 1995: 311)

Research does support claims that refraining from ever smoking or giving up smoking is associated with lowering the risk of developing a number of diseases such as lung cancer, cardiovascular disease and stroke. Other studies also suggest that lifestyle behaviours such as not drinking alcohol to excess, eating a nutritious diet and partaking in exercise are associated with a decrease in mortality from certain diseases (Puska 1985; Imperial Cancer Research Fund OXCHECK Study 1995; Elley *et al.* 2003). Some authors argue that 'an over reliance on epidemiology in developing health promotion programmes manifests itself also in the definition of desirable outcomes' (Tannahill 1992: 99). Thus evaluations of lifestyle change programmes have focused too narrowly on mortality and morbidity statistics and neglected other outcomes such as increased social networks, educational outcomes and people's feelings and experiences.

It is widely believed that a healthy lifestyle results in improvements in less tangible health outcomes such as a sense of wellbeing, improved energy and physical fitness.

Lifestyle-focused health promotion has been embraced by many social groups (for example, women, the elderly, community nurses, social workers and some ethnic communities) because they welcome the potential of community-based disease prevention to reduce inequalities of health and death (Taylor and Ford 1981; Foster 1995; Williams and Calnan 1996). For example, Oakley (1989) found that while large-scale public health attempts to encourage women to stop smoking when pregnant are unsuccessful, small-scale community-based programmes which offer women social and infrastructure support do result in a reduction in smoking and improved self-esteem and social conditions for the women involved.

However, many other studies show contradictory results. For example, an epidemiological study of middle-aged men found that in comparison with a control group, the mortality rates were higher for those men who had been randomly selected to participate in cholesterol-lowering and exercise programmes (Strandberg *et al.* 1991). A nationally representative prospective study of 3,617 American adults reached the conclusion that while reducing health risk behaviours such as smoking and drinking would improve the health of Americans, the differences in mortality between people of low socio-economic status and those of high socio-economic status are due to a wide array of factors including education and income, and '[t]hese differences would persist even with improved health behaviours among the disadvantaged' (Lantz *et al.* 1998: 1703).

The effectiveness of individually focused lifestyle interventions has been cast into considerable doubt by a recent systematic review and meta-analysis of randomised controlled trials of multiple risk factor interventions for preventing coronary disease conducted by two professors of clinical epidemiology, Shah Ebrahim and George Davey Smith (Ebrahim and Davey Smith 1997, 2000). This study is presented as a 1997 article in the *British Medical Journal* and as a Cochrane Database review in 2000. Ebrahim and Davey Smith examined a total of eighteen trials from around the world and conducted a complex statistical analysis to investigate the 'effects of multiple risk factor intervention for reducing cardiovascular risk factors, total mortality and mortality from coronary heart disease among adults without clinical evidence of established cardiovascular disease' (Ebrahim and Davey Smith 2000: CD001561). They found that in the general population, counselling, education and drug treatments were 'ineffective in achieving reduction in total mortality or mortality from cardiovascular disease' (1997: 1666). While the authors did find a reduction in mortality and risk factors in trials focused on reducing hypertension, these trials were most successful when they involved people needing control of hypertension and cholesterol. These trials also used drug treatments in addition to lifestyle counselling. Overall the authors reported that:

> The pooled effects suggest multiple risk factor intervention has no effect on mortality and risk factor effects were relatively modest, and were related to the amount of pharmacological treatment used, and in some cases may have been over-estimated because of regression to mean effects, lack of intention to treat analyses, habituation to blood pressure measurement, and the use of self reports of smoking. . . . The evidence suggests that such interventions have limited utility in the general population.
>
> (Ebrahim and Davey Smith 2000: CD001561)

In their conclusions Ebrahim and Davey Smith commented on several important issues related to lifestyle modification-focused health promotion. First, they state that the more successful interventions reviewed in their study would 'far exceed what is feasible in routine practice' (1997: 1468) and also that the small results found in their analysis seem inefficient given the 'huge resources' put into the trials in terms of money, expertise and time. The authors conclude by recommending a shift in focus from lifestyle counselling as the disease prevention method of choice for general populations to a greater recognition of the importance of fiscal, legislative and structural measures aimed at reducing smoking, creating opportunities for exercise and increasing access to nutritious foods. In an editorial published in the *British Medical Journal* Ebrahim *et al.* (2000) also suggest retargeting risk-modifying efforts aiming to reduce deaths from cardiovascular disease by using secondary prevention and targeting high-risk groups.

In addition to querying the health outcomes of lifestyle modification, the ability of health promotion programmes to actually produce modifications of people's lifestyles has also been questioned (Mechanic 1994; Stott *et al.*

1994). Critics argue that such programmes have only a limited capacity to produce lifestyle changes because they rely almost entirely on health education about lifestyle risks rather than addressing the cultural or structural issues which underlie lifestyle behaviours and practices (Byde 1989; Beattie 1991; Mechanic 1994). Certainly the ability of educational and counselling interventions to achieve sustained risk factor-altering lifestyle modification appears doubtful. A systematic review of long-term outcomes from interventions consisting of advice to reduce dietary salt in adults found that only very 'intensive interventions unsuited to primary care or population prevention programmes' produced longer-term change and even these provided 'only small reductions in blood pressure and sodium excretion, and effects on deaths or cardiovascular events are unclear' (Hooper *et al.* 2002: 628). Several studies suggest that some groups such as families of heart disease patients, school children and retired people appear to be amenable to lifestyle modification (Calfas *et al.* 1996; Higginbotham *et al.* 1999). However, even among those people willing to change, longer-term behavioural change is rare (Van Beurden *et al.* 1993; Jacobs *et al.* 2004). There are many barriers to conscious long-term behavioural change for the purpose of reducing health risks (Mechanic 1994; Ritchie *et al.* 1994). Furthermore, the relationship between behavioural change and changes in biological risk factors such as body mass index or blood pressure is variable. For example, one of the few studies that did appear to show significant behavioural changes lasting over a twelve-month period also found that 'behaviour changes were not translated into differences in biological risk factors' (Steptoe *et al.* 1999: 944).

In addition, it appears that health professionals do not enjoy providing lifestyle counselling or receiving it (this is explored in detail in the next section of this chapter). In summary, studies of the attitudes towards lifestyle education and counselling for the purpose of disease prevention show that doctors find this activity to be dull and time consuming and they are doubtful about its usefulness (e.g. Toon 1995; Williams and Calnan 1994). Furthermore, many patients also do not appear to enjoy lifestyle counselling. While lay people consider that disease prevention is important they don't like being told what to do or being made to feel guilty about their actions (e.g. Stott and Pill 1990; Stott *et al.* 1994). Patients' reluctance to undergo lifestyle counselling is also supported by well-documented problems in recruiting patients (and health care practitioners) to intervention studies (e.g. Steptoe *et al.* 1999).

Critics of lifestyle counselling and education claim that the failure of such health promotion programmes is well documented and well recognised but that the programmes remain popular because they make governments look authoritative and active, while at the same time avoiding confrontations that might prove politically costly (Lupton 1995; Petersen 1996; Richmond 2002). Florin (1999) reviewed the development and implementation of prevention strategies in the 1990 GP contract in the UK. She found that the 'popularity and cheapness of the health check approach, rather than research findings, were most influential in the rise of health checks and the development of the 1990 health promotion contract' (Florin 1999: 1274).

It also appears to be the case that many of the researchers trialling these interventions are deeply committed to a lifestyle approach. Studies reporting small or no changes in behaviours often continue to recommend lifestyle counselling as a disease prevention measure, suggesting that if their trial could not measure changes they need new measurement instruments or simply to work even harder on achieving success. For example, Tudor-Smith *et al.* (1998) report the final results from a community-based demonstration programme named Heartbeat Wales designed to modify behavioural risks for cardiovascular disease. The authors report that no definite conclusions could be drawn concerning the efficacy of the programme (treatment and matched reference groups showed similar changes in behaviours such as smoking rates). However, the authors then suggest that new 'evaluation techniques need to be developed' so that the success of such programmes can be measured effectively (1998: 822). Similarly, Steptoe *et al.* (1999) found that after a programme involving intensive counselling from nurses and reported changes in behavioural risk factors for cardiovascular disease, their research subjects showed no change in biological risk factors (with the exception of systolic blood pressure). In response, Steptoe *et al.* (1999) suggest that extending the amount and intensity of counselling by practice nurses may be necessary to translate behavioural change into 'measurable reductions in risk'.

In addition to highlighting the limited ability of lifestyle education and counselling to produce improvements in health outcomes or to achieve long-term lifestyle change, the sociological critique has identified a number of other problems arising from health promotion focused on lifestyle modification. These include the 'worried well' phenomenon and associated increases in health care consumption and unexpected responses to health promotion messages.

The term worried well has been used in medical literature since the early 1980s to describe apparently healthy individuals who make frequent medical visits (Smith *et al.* 2002). Typically the worried well are described as expensive malingerers. As discussed in the previous chapter, health promotion and the new public health are associated with a widespread increase in concern about health risks (Crawford 1980; Beck 1990; Lupton 1995). As Fitzpatrick writes, 'We live in strange times. People in Western society live longer and healthier lives than ever before. Yet people seem increasingly preoccupied by their health' (2001: 1). Mass advertising campaigns about health risks and health promotion campaigns advocating screening and lifestyle modification in order to prevent disease have increased the numbers of healthy people who are worried about the state of their health and who seek reassurance from medical visits and testing. This rather logical consequence of risk factor health promotion has been viewed with considerable concern by health promoters and the medical profession.

> People no longer seem to view their state of health in a light hearted manner. The worried well hunger for every scrap of information they can find about their physical well-being, with the result that a veritable diagnostic industry is developing.
>
> (Giard 2003: 1893)

Fylkesnes and Førde (1993a, 1993b) and Førde (1998) claim that risk factor health promotion has led to a cultural change resulting in increased consumption of health care resources and increased anxiety. Ironically, in many cases the people who are classified as high risk for certain disease have not increased their doctor visits or requests for screening while those at low risk have (Van Beurden *et al.* 1993; Dozier *et al.* 1997).

In addition, lifestyle-focused health promotion campaigns sometimes produce an unexpected or negative response (e.g. Crawford 1978; Kelly and Charlton 1992; Stott *et al.* 1994), quite different to those intended by health promoters or health care professionals. As described above, one response is an increase in fear and anxiety about health. However, unlike the response of the worried well, that is increased demand for screening tests, certain groups of people appear to interpret lifestyle messages in terms of self-blame and fear of blame from others. This may in turn lead to a reluctance to seek medical care for symptoms such as chest pain or chronic cough. For example, Richards *et al.* (2003) investigated possible negative effects of life-style advice related to cardiovascular disease. They conducted interviews with thirty Glaswegians (fifteen men and fifteen women), drawn equally from a socio-economically deprived area and from an affluent area. They found that:

> Respondents recognised the causative links between well-established cardiac risk factor and heart disease. Individuals blamed themselves for their heart disease and general ill health and many also believed that they would be blamed for their behaviour and health problems by doctors. For some respondents, self-blame and fear of blame appeared to contribute to a reluctance to seek care. Self-blame, experience of blame and fear of blame were more common in respondents from deprived areas.
>
> (Richard *et al.* 2003: 711)

Another way in which health promotion messages may not produce their intended outcome is when they are subverted or transgressed by the recipients (Frankel *et al.* 1991; Lawler *et al.* 2003; Baska *et al.* 2004). Lay epidemiology may compete with medical discourses about the causes of disease and preventive health, leading to either very different interpretations of the meaning of health promotion messages or scepticism about health promotion information (Davison *et al.* 1991, 1992; Frankel *et al.* 1991). Crossley (2002, 2004) describes this process using two quite different examples. The first concerns 'barebacking', a term used by some gay men to describe sex without a condom. This practice is seen as unsafe sex as it increases the risks of HIV infection and other sexually transmitted diseases. Despite the early success of health promotion in educating gay men about the importance of condoms rates of usage are falling and young gay men in particular appear to be resisting the safe sex message. Crossley examined published narratives from gay men and found that 'contemporary "bare-backing" behaviour may constitute one manifestation of "resistance" or "transgressional habitus" that has remained a consistent feature of gay men's individual and social psyche since the early days of gay liberation' (2004: 225). She also found that for young gay men condom use was associated with the practices of older men and was seen as giving less intimate sex. In her second example Crossley (2002) analysed responses from a focus group of members of a Women's Institute in a northern British city. During a discussion about health promotion several women discussed smoking cessation and health education leaflets. She found the women joked about not wanting to read the leaflets provided on the table and mocked the information contained in them by reading from them in a deliberately playful manner. One of the women who described herself as a committed cigarette smoker also changed a conversation on the importance of smoking cessation by telling a joke, saying it 'wouldn't make any difference' and discussing the importance of pleasure in life. Crossley describes this as an 'excellent behavioural example of resistance to health promotion' (2002: 1478).

If the medical approach to lifestyle has proved to be less than successful in the realm of public health, epidemiology and health promotion, has it been more successful for individual medical practitioners and their patients?

Is lifestyle counselling effective in medical consultations?

There are a small number of studies which investigate doctors' understandings of lifestyle and how these are applied during medical consultations. The majority of these studies maintain the focus on preventive health/health promotion found in other sociological writing about lifestyle. They also suggest that doctors do not find lifestyle-focused health promotion easy to convey during medical consultations, that there is considerable variation in the ways that individual doctors understand and 'make sense' of lifestyle as a explanatory concept and that doctors and their patients recognise a number of negative consequences that may arise when explaining the causes and prevention of disease in terms of lifestyle (Sackett 2002; Getz *et al.* 2003).

These studies can be divided into two groups. The first investigates practice. A number of these have involved observing or audio-recording doctor/patient conversations about prevention, often in the context of a general practice consultation (Beaudoin *et al.* 2001). Others have used questionnaires to survey doctors and (at times also practice nurses) about health promotion activities using lifestyle counselling (e.g. Laitakari *et al.* 1997; McKenna and Vernon 2004). The second group of studies explores the views of doctors (and sometimes patients) about the use of lifestyle advice and counselling during medical consultations as a disease prevention activity.

Studies investigating practice have produced mixed findings about the frequency with which doctors talked about lifestyle during a consultation. Boulton and Williams (1983) and Tuckett *et al.* (1985) found that prevention is not a dominant feature of doctor/patient consultations. However, others such as Tapper-Jones (1986), Stott and Pill (1990), Johanson *et al.* (1994) and McKenna and Vernon (2004) argue that including discussion of prevention in the consultation is a growing trend and a reflection of the widespread acceptance of health promotion and health education throughout the community. For example, Johanson *et al.* (1994) found that talking about lifestyle matters took up one-third of the total consultation time spent in doctor/patient dialogue. However, the authors included time spent by doctors listening and supporting patients while they spoke about a broad range of issues including family, work and relationships. The majority of the time classified as lifestyle discussion was spent in talking in this way, rather than in counselling patients to modify their lifestyles in specific ways to prevent specific diseases. Johanson *et al.* (1998), in a study of forty-two audio-recorded consultations (between general practitioners and their patients in Sweden), also found that doctors were using much broader conceptions of lifestyle than those commonly found in health promotion. They asked about structural issues such as housing and work, issues relating to family, work and romantic relationships, issues related to environmental toxins and advice related to individual measures such as alcohol, smoking, diet and exercise (Johanson *et al.* 1998: 105). Johanson *et al.* also found that while doctors talked about lifestyle and prevention a great deal, they carefully avoided 'making explicit medical inferences about specific issues concerning the individual's lifestyle' (1998: 103). The authors suggest that by not sharing their detailed knowledge about relationships between lifestyle issues and health, the doctors are depriving patients of valuable opportunities to improve their health. In contrast, the doctors they interviewed claimed that they avoided making specific associations between their patients' lifestyles and their illnesses for fear of negative reactions to such advice.

Johanson *et al.* (1998) also found that doctors use discussion about lifestyle quite differently from their patients. Physicians use lifestyle information in a relatively systematic way as a resource in clinical reasoning. Talking to a patient about lifestyle helps doctors to decide which medical issues might be pertinent for each individual. Patients, on the other hand, use lifestyle advice to define their identity or to elicit certain medical treatments.

Beaudoin *et al.* (2001) conducted a similar study in Canada. They audiotaped consultations by thirty-five family physicians (equivalent to a general practitioner) with 148 patients. They conducted a statistical analysis of these data and found that the doctors frequently spoke briefly about weight, diet, nutrition, physical activity and tobacco use. 'On average, the visits contained discussion of 3.6 different issues for a total time of 2.9 minutes' (2001: 275). Female doctors or patients seen to have a poorer mental health status were both associated with more frequent use of lifestyle conversation. However, the authors also found that while lifestyle discussion was frequent, it was limited in scope and tended to be most common in consultations with targeted patients.

Studies investigating doctors' views on lifestyle as an explanatory concept for disease prevention became popular in the 1980s and 1990s as government policies in the UK, Australia, New Zealand and Canada and professional medical groups such as the Colleges of General Practitioners advocated the use of lifestyle counselling and advice by doctors as a means of modifying patient risk factors and supporting healthy lifestyles. In Australia, for example, GPs are advised to identify patients at risk, assess the level of risk factor and then provide written information, a lifestyle prescription, brief advice and motivational interviewing in addition to other forms of assistance such as pharmacotherapies and referral (RACGP SNAP Guidelines 2004). However, a number of studies show that there may be a 'considerable discrepancy between the rhetoric of prevention as espoused by the Government and professional bodies such as the Royal College of General Practitioners alike, and the reality of prevention and health promotion at a grass-roots level within general practice' (Williams and Calnan 1994: 373). A number of researchers have investigated this issue including Williams (1983), Williams and Boulton (1988), Tuckett *et al.* (1985), Tapper-Jones (1986), Coulter (1987), Boulton and Williams (1986), Williams and Calnan (1994) and McKinlay *et al.* (2005). Most of these researchers produced similar findings, which is remarkable considering that these studies span a twenty-year period and draw on GPs from different geographic locations and with very different working conditions and practice populations.

What they all found was that many doctors, about one in three in one of the earliest studies, were doubtful about the usefulness of social intervention into disease. In so far as they were concerned about prevention they 'conceptualised [preventive health] solely in terms of compliance in order to exercise firmer control over the management of disease and patient' (Willams and Boulton 1988: 237). These doctors and many of the doctors in a later study (Willams and Calnan 1994) found lifestyle counselling boring, time consuming and a distraction from curative medicine. Many were also sceptical about the evidence for the relationship between lifestyle and disease. As one doctor said when asked to describe a coronary candidate, 'They are all fat, smoke like chimneys and generally lie around. But I have hundreds of these and they never have heart attacks' (Williams and Calnan 1996: 383).

Other doctors were also worried that health education and health promotion conveyed hidden messages that were not altogether desirable. By seeking to increase awareness of health and healthy living, some believed they could also create anxiety, dependence and a restricted life. Associated with these concerns, several doctors said that health promotion and education were 'essentially intrusive and moralistic' (Williams and Boulton 1988: 242). They believed this to be 'at odds with the GP's role as morally neutral and technically specific' (Williams and Boulton 1988: 242).

Some doctors, however, were fully committed to producing lifestyle change in their patients. These doctors saw '[disease] prevention mainly as a form of intervention on lifestyle and risk factors ... they had a clear idea of its aims, as promoting behaviour change in individual patients and encouraging greater self-care' (Williams and Boulton 1988: 239). This group of doctors placed considerable emphasis on patient education, the importance of personal motivation in behaviour change and their own personal commitment to prevention. This included taking a moral stand in the community and revealing their own habits to influence their patients.

It seems clear from these studies that GPs are not a united group when it comes to their views about using lifestyle as an orientating concept for disease prevention and health promotion. All of the studies cited found variations between GPs in terms of their attitudes towards lifestyle counselling in their consultations. Despite this variation, however, GPs across a twenty-year period seem to share many common concerns related to explaining certain diseases in terms of individual lifestyle behaviours and to hold serious doubts about the practicalities and usefulness of providing lifestyle advice to their patients in an effort to prevent disease.

Conclusion

From the 1970s until the mid-1980s much sociological writing about lifestyle focused on disease prevention and epidemiology was positive (e.g. Kickbusch 1986b; Russell and Buisson 1988; Badura and Kickbusch 1991). Medical attempts to explain health and disease using a social model were seen by sociologists as commendable, and as recognition of longstanding sociological arguments about the social patterning of health and disease (Mant 1989). In contrast, throughout the mid-1980s, 1990s and early 2000s, a body of sociological writing emerged which was highly critical of medical understandings of lifestyle, particularly as represented by epidemiology and public health. This coincided with an increased focus within these fields on individual risk factors and a move away from population and structural factors as causes of disease and poor health. Pearce describes this as 'a shift in the level of analysis from the population to the individual' (1996: 678).

Sociological concern about risk factor epidemiology, lifestyle-focused health promotion and the increasingly individualist focus of public health is a reflection of fundamental differences between sociological and epidemiological understandings of what constitutes a social explanation for disease.

In sum, sociological criticism of the lifestyle approach found in epidemiology, aspects of the new public health and risk factor health promotion argues that individualist and risk factor understandings of lifestyle are fundamentally flawed as explanatory concepts for health and illness. The relationship between individual lifestyle behaviours and disease is uncertain. The usefulness of lifestyle change as a means of reducing morbidity and mortality is questionable. Furthermore, health promotion aiming to produce modification of people's lifestyles through education campaigns has a low success rate in terms of producing long-term behavioural changes.

As discussed in chapter 1, within public health these criticisms have resulted in a reconceptualisation of health promotion to include a wider focus on the environment (psychological, social and physical) as seen in the new public health. However, such reconceptualisation has not changed the way that epidemiological research is conducted or, apparently, the ways that such research is interpreted by those within public health: 'Despite murmurings at the international level in support of changing environments, most health promotion activity in Western countries such as Australia has continued to be narrowly focused around educating people to change their lifestyles' (Richmond 1997: 158).

Furthermore, the expansion of a lifestyle approach to include the environment has not become practice in many countries and may not alleviate the problems associated with a reductive lifestyle approach. Finally, it may add a range of new, potentially negative implications due to issues such as victim blaming, an expanded health concept and an increased scope for public health (Petersen and Lupton 1996). These issues are explored in detail in the following chapter. Nor are medical understandings of a lifestyle approach successful in the context of medical consultations. Studies of GPs suggest that doctors find lifestyle-focused health promotion difficult to apply in their work. They are also aware of potentially negative consequences for their patients such as increased anxiety, self-blame and confusion.

3 Assumptions underlying the medical approach to lifestyle

Introduction

In addition to questioning the efficacy of medical conceptions of lifestyle as an orientating framework for disease prevention, sociologists have also expressed concern about many of the assumptions underlying a lifestyle approach and the implications of these for people who become unwell (e.g. Crawford 1978, 1980; Bunton and Macdonald 1992; Lupton 1993; Nettleton and Bunton 1995). This cultural critique is the second aspect of the wider sociological critique of a lifestyle approach. Like the arguments about the usefulness of medical ideas about lifestyle for disease prevention programmes outlined in the previous chapter, medical understandings of lifestyle have largely been addressed by sociologists in the context of health promotion, epidemiology and public health.

Contemporary medical understandings of lifestyle, health and disease have attracted sociological interest and critique because they have a range of important implications both for those who are being understood and for those who are striving to understand. As a medical explanatory framework, lifestyle is heavily laden with cultural baggage. The most frequently described of these cultural burdens are that lifestyle understandings are moralistic and discriminatory, that they increase the potential for medicalisation, medical surveillance and medical control, that they reflect, reinforce and reproduce contemporary concerns with the management and containment of risks, that they are associated with commodifying and commercialising the body and health, and that despite claims of being an alternative to traditional medical approaches to disease they actually reflect a continuation and expansion of modernist and science-based medical explanation.

Each of these arguments is discussed in detail in this chapter, commencing with the argument that a lifestyle approach has a tendency to blame the victim and is thus moralistic and potentially discriminatory.

Moralistic and discriminatory

Models of disease that place responsibility for illness on individuals and the wider ideology of lifestylism are both fundamentally moral. 'Once health is linked with virtue, then the regulation of lifestyle in the name of health becomes a mechanism for deterring vice and disciplining society as a whole' (Fitzpatrick 2001: 8). The underlying premise of a lifestyle approach is that 'good' behaviour will keep people healthy and that 'bad' behaviour will make them sick. A healthy life is viewed as a virtuous life and illness suggests a failure to live a virtuous life. This phenomenon is often termed 'victim blaming'. Disease or poor health is conceptualised in terms of individuals' non-compliance with the rules of a healthy lifestyle (Sontag 1989; Richardson 1991; Epstein 1995; Greco 1993):

> when risk is believed to be internally imposed because of lack of willpower, moral weakness or laziness on the part of the individual the reciprocal relationship of sin and risk is reversed. Those who are deemed to be 'at risk' become sinners, not the sinned against, because of their apparent voluntary courting of risk.
>
> (Lupton 1995: 90)

Fitzpatrick, a British GP highly critical of the new public health and healthism, argues that under the lifestyle approach 'disease states are increasingly evaluated in psychological or moral terms' (2001: 6). He suggests that the obscure nature of many lifestyle diseases has left the realm of explanation open to the view that 'people become sick because they want to (as for example in the view that cancer results from "stress" or "depression") or because they deserve to (because they smoke or drink too much)' (2001: 6).

An explanatory perspective that explains disease in terms of lifestyle is particularly problematic for those people who develop a disease or condition held to be the direct result of something they did or did not do in their daily living (Horton and Aggleton 1989). This is demonstrated in some studies investigating lay beliefs about the causes of disease such as cardiovascular disease or cancer. For example, Richards *et al.* (2003) found that interview respondents described feeling responsible and guilty about chest pain while Ryan and Skinner (1999) found that first-degree relatives of breast cancer patients said that lifestyle factors contribute to breast cancer risk and that they thought they could reduce their personal risk through lifestyle modification. Susan Sontag has also described the way in which widespread beliefs about the moral nature of disease and notions of individual responsibility for certain diseases led to feelings of guilt and self-blame for tuberculosis patients, cancer patients and people affected by HIV/AIDS (Sontag 1978, 1989).

The explicit morality of a lifestyle approach contrasts with the construction of disease categories in other medical approaches (such as germ theory or genetic models of disease). While these are recognised as also having implicit moral bases, such approaches appear on the surface to be value-free. For example, in germ theory, disease is seen to result from factors external to the individual (e.g. bacteria or viruses) and in genetic models of disease ill-health is associated with genetic defects and generally seen as being outside the control of individuals.

The moral nature of a lifestyle approach is potentially discriminatory in a number of different ways. Healthy people who are seen to be damaging their health through their behaviours may be discriminated against by insurance companies or employers (Bunton *et al.* 1995; Bunton and Burrows 1995). For example, smokers and overweight people are frequently asked to pay higher insurance premiums. People already in poor health due to lifestyle-related conditions may be refused certain medical treatments, for example organ transplants or drug trials, if they continue their 'unhealthy' behaviours (Davison and Davey Smith 1995; Mackie *et al.* 2001).

Another discriminatory aspect of an individualised lifestyle approach is that such an approach implies blame even though lifestyle risks are not equally distributed across the community. To act as though they are or as though exposure to lifestyle risks is entirely the result of individual choice, as in risk factor health promotion, is discriminatory (Leichter 2003). Structural, behavioural and psychosocial determinants of health vary accord-ing to factors such as gender, geography, age, ethnicity and occupation (Brimblecombe *et al.* 2000; Denton *et al.* 2004; Leyland 2004; Irabarren *et al.* 2005). Members of low-income groups experience exclusion and lack of control over their lives. Failure to recognise the links between material conditions and health-related risks is dishonest, unfair and pointless in terms of disease prevention (Davison *et al.* 1991; Blackburn 1992; Naidoo and Wills 1998).

For example, certain groups in Australia, in particular the socio-economically disadvantaged and Aboriginal Australians, have higher rates of lifestyle risks for a number of diseases, in particular cardiovascular dis-ease, stroke and diabetes (Australian Institute of Health and Welfare 2002). In the UK unemployed people and the elderly often eat diets low in nutrition (Widgery 1993). They are also more likely to have cold or damp housing and experience difficulties in participating in physical activity and accessing primary care (Connelly and Crown 1994).

Another lifestyle risk factor that shows very clear differences according to age, socio-economic status, gender, occupation and education is cigarette smoking. Despite a general decline in smoking rates in many countries, rates of smoking remain higher among disadvantaged people and they seem to find smoking cessation more difficult (Kemm 2001). Some authors have suggested this is because smoking is a prop and coping strategy for people living in a challenging social environment (Bancroft *et al.* 2003). Social gradients in smoking have also become more apparent over time in the UK (Jefferis *et al.* 2004). Smoking rates are also patterned according to gender and occupation. In the mid- to late twentieth century more men than women took up smoking. However, men have stopped smoking in larger numbers than women and young women are taking up smoking at higher rates than men. Some occupational groups such as nurses and manual workers also have higher smoking rates than others such as doctors or office workers (Marang-van de Mheen *et al.* 1999; Pearce 1996; Blaxter 1990).

Morbidity and mortality rates are also higher among the disadvantaged. However, despite clear evidence of social patterns in the distribution of risk factors, the lifestyle approach continues to position lifestyle risks as individual responsibilities and choices. Thus the members of such groups risk being blamed for their poor health and being seen as dangerous to others (Davis and George 1990; Nettleton 1995; Petersen and Lupton 1996).

The complexities surrounding the relationships between morality, social location and lifestyle risks can be seen in the example of women's exercise. Women have lower rates of physical activity than similarly aged men (Fullagar 2002). Increasing the physical activity levels of women is a focus in many health promotion campaigns as these have changed little over the last thirty years. Willis has shown that contemporary exercise ideology which represents physical exercise for women as socially acceptable is 'a recent victory in women's struggle for equality for men' (1991: 65). However, he and other authors also argue that the current focus on enhancing women's health through exercise ignores inequities which range from socio-economic inequality, the continued medicalisation of the female body, the emphasis on women's physical appearance, stereotypes of women related to motherhood, ageing, menstruation and menopause and issues of diversity and race (Vertinsky 1998; Love *et al.* 1997; Lewis and Ridge 2005). Vertinsky (1998) contends that the low rates of female participation in exercise should not be seen as a reflection of poor self-discipline or lack of knowledge about the health benefits of exercise; instead they should be understood as the manifestation of a lack of opportunities to either participate in exercise or to enjoy exercise as a result of social, political, economic and cultural gender inequality (Vertinsky 1998).

Lewis and Ridge (2005) demonstrate the ways in which being a mother to young children makes physical exercise a complex issue for women. They conducted a qualitative study with forty Australian mothers of children under six. Their findings show that the way women think about exercise and the reasons why they would see it as a positive and healthy activity differ from those often described in risk factor health promotion. They also highlight that women are very aware of ' "troubling social discourses" surrounding exercise and motherhood' (2005: 2304). Women were aware of stereotypes of maternal obligation and the discourses surrounding being a 'superwoman'. They also felt uneasy about cultural pressures to have a slim and controlled body. Reconciling these issues with health promotion messages about activity and health was difficult for the women. However, they also expressed a desire to participate in pleasurable activities and to be active.

Our study indicates that health promotion messages which emphasise individual health and fitness over the collective interests of family friendship networks and community are unlikely to resonate with the way mothers of young children understand the role of physical activity in their lives ... for young mothers physical activity is considered 'healthy' when it strengthens women's relationships and identities as mothers.

(Lewis and Ridge 2005: 2305)

The discrimination which flows from a lifestyle approach can be either overt, as mentioned above in relation to increased insurance premiums for smokers, or covert, in the sense that well-intended health promotion programmes inadvertently help to 'reproduce structures of inequality in relation to dominance' (White *et al.* 1995: 161).

Expanding the health concept, medicalisation and surveillance

Critiques of a lifestyle approach which refer to the expansion of the concept of health, medicalisation and surveillance are linked by a concern with the ways in which a lifestyle approach has led to changes in the way health is understood and the perceived relationship between medicine and health. A lifestyle approach to explaining disease and health is associated with an expanded health concept and an increase in concern about perceived threats to health that is sometimes termed healthism (see Nettleton 1995; Førde 1998). The number of factors or aspects of life seen as being related to health are much greater from within a biopsychosocial lifestyle approach. Unlike the traditional medical model of disease where understandings are limited to physical aberrations from 'normal', the focus on risk, future disease and individual behaviours means that under a lifestyle approach almost every aspect of living is seen as health related, for example food, leisure, sun exposure, clothing, sex life, social relationships, housing, drug use and physical activity. Furthermore, increased concern about health means that these aspects of everyday life become problematised. Thus not only are many more behaviours and practices now viewed as health related but they also become worrying and defined in terms of their relationship towards either damaging health or promoting and maintaining health. For example, in Australia leisure time is no longer seen simply as time away from work where individuals engage in pleasurable activity. Instead, leisure is viewed as a time for health-promoting physical activity (Fullagar 2002). Even if the activities remain the same, their meaning has changed to one related to maintaining and promoting health. Such an expanded health concept has been linked by sociologists with processes of medicalisation and surveillance.

The term medicalisation has come to refer to the complex process by which medicine is judged to be the appropriate social institution to deal with issues of disease and sickness. An increasingly large number of social issues come to be defined as illnesses or disorders and thus as medical problems. These social issues now defined as medical problems come under medical governance, are described in medical language, understood in terms of a medical framework and managed through medical intervention (Fox 1977; Conrad and Schneider 1980; Conrad 1992). Examples of these processes are 'states of being' that have become included in the sphere of medical concern including life stages such as adolescence or old age, life events such as childbirth or pregnancy, behaviours and practices such as alcoholism, fasting or bingeing and masturbation. Promiscuity, sadness, homosexuality and obesity have all at times been defined as disease states (Freidson 1970; Chessler 1972; Zola 1972; Fox 1989; Lowenberg and Davis 1994). A recent addition to this list is ADHD (Attention Deficit Hyperactivity Disorder); this conceptualises some childhood behaviours as a disease syndrome to be treated by drugs such as Ritalin (Singh 2004).

Conrad and Schneider (1980) consider that medicalisation can occur on a number of levels: first, at the conceptual level, when medical vocabulary is used to define a problem, for example 'postnatal depression'; second, at the institutional level, when an institution achieves medical legitimacy, for example physiotherapy or dietetics; third, at the level of the doctor/patient relationship, when the doctor defines problems as being medical through the process of diagnosis and treatment.

Medicalisation is generally perceived by medical sociologists as a negative process (Lupton 1997). Some writers have expressed concern about the increasing power of the medical profession throughout the twentieth century and the problems associated with medicine replacing religion or the family as a major agent of social control (e.g. Freidson 1970; Zola 1972; Conrad and Schneider 1980; Martin 1987). Other authors have argued that medicalisation should be viewed non-judgementally as a process which can be helpful in some contexts and destructive in others (Lowenberg and Davis 1994; Broom and Woodward 1996).

Understanding disease and health in terms of lifestyle has the potential to increase medicalisation in two ways. The preventive focus on currently healthy people who might become unwell in the future increases the sphere of medical concern from states of illness to include health (Fitzgerald 1994; Hughes 1994). Contemporary medical notions of lifestyle risk, where all people are required to consider their risk of disease even when they are currently healthy, puts bodies into a state of transition where health is transformed into 'virtual disease' (Hughes 1994: 57). Furthermore, if medicine is utilising an approach towards disease that focuses on the social rather than only the biological, the self-limitation imposed by the biological reductionism of germ theory (the medical model) is removed and the sphere of possible medical influence is further increased. Lowenberg and Davis (1994) term this process, whereby the range of factors considered to be of importance to medicine is increased, an expansion of the pathogenic sphere.

Medical sociologists who adopt a Foucauldian perspective have focused on the body 'as a target of disciplinary practices' (Turner 1996: 21) and extended the medicalisation critique to argue that a lifestyle approach as articulated through 'the programmes and technologies of health promotion' has contributed to 'an increasingly all encompassing network of surveillance and observation' (Nettleton and Bunton 1995: 47). These authors draw on Foucault's writings about disciplinary power and panoptic surveillance to examine 'the ways in which forms of governance involve the investigation and regulation of the body of the individual and bodies of populations' (Nettleton and Bunton 1995: 47). The disciplinary power of medicine involves the strategies of 'observation, examination, measurement and the comparison of individuals against an established norm, bringing them into a field of visibility' (Lupton 1997: 99).

There are two aspects to the surveillance critique. The first focuses on how the popularity of lifestyle discourses reflects a displacement of the traditional medical site of surveillance, the clinic, by the discursive space of epidemiology and the related technologies of health promotion and health education. This is 'symbolised through a strategic shift to the psycho-social dimensions of disease and the spatio-temporal calculus of risk, crystallised in the new emphasis on "lifestyles" ' (Williams 2001: 148). In this argument the disciplinary powers of medicine have been increased by medical adoption of a lifestyle approach or what Armstrong calls 'social medicine' (Armstrong 1983: 38–40). Disease prevention measures which focus on lifestyle are viewed by these authors as evidence of the 'growing penetration of the clinical gaze into the everyday lives of citizens, including their emotional states, the nature of their interpersonal relationships, the management of stress and other "lifestyle" choices' (Lupton 1997: 107). An emphasis on monitoring population risk factors and the capacity of technological advances to achieve sophisticated 'systematic pre-detection' is seen to legitimate new modes of surveillance (Bunton and Burrows 1995: 209).

The surveillance argument also recognises how the disciplinary powers of medicine have expanded state involvement in profiling, monitoring and regulating populations (Arney and Bergen 1984; Armstrong 1993). Governments working with neo-liberal political ideologies and concerned about ageing populations and rising health costs play a key role in promoting and maintaining the popularity and dominance of a lifestyle approach. 'Risk discourse in the public health sphere serves the political function of allowing the state, as owners of knowledge, to exert power over the bodies of its citizens' (Lupton 1994a: 138). For example, in addition to the clear relationship between the state and medicine as evidenced by state-run public health and health promotion programmes, individual doctors and nurses are often dependent on government funding which is conditional on their becoming 'health strategists' (Nettleton and Bunton 1995: 48). In many instances one of these conditions is that health professionals apply a lifestyle approach to disease prevention. For example, the British GP contracts in the early 1990s encouraged GPs to engage in disease prevention activities such as lifestyle counselling and exercise prescriptions (Fitzpatrick 2001). This disease prevention strategy is now being used in Australia and New Zealand (McKinlay *et al.* 2005). States also promote a lifestyle approach through the allocation of research funds. For example, in terms of epidemiological and public health research, priority areas in Australia clearly emphasise the importance of disease prevention for conditions such as diabetes and arthritis. They also emphasise the importance of identifying and monitoring risk factors such as obesity and high blood pressure. Thus research investigating these issues is more likely to be funded through the National Health and Medical Research Council scheme.

The second aspect of the surveillance critique addresses the 'interrelationship between the imperatives of bodily management expressed at the institutional level and ways that individuals engage in the conduct of everyday life' (Lupton 1997: 103). Because a lifestyle approach to disease prevention places emphasis on self-control, self-discipline and self-monitoring of lifestyle risks, surveillance is carried out by individuals as they assess their own bodies, states of health or sickness and ways of living in terms of medical/public health advice about lifestyle (Glassner 1989; Lupton 1994a; Dean 1999).

Thus the surveillance critique focuses on the ways that a lifestyle-focused approach to disease prevention has several components and the implications of these for disciplinary power (Turner 1996; Nettleton and Bunton 1995). This critique also focuses on relationships between the state, the medical profession and individuals when disease prevention is conceptualised in terms of self-regulation and the 'creation of the health promoting self' (Nettleton 1995: 47).

Commodification and consumer culture

Advanced capitalist societies have been described as having a consumer culture (Bourdieu 1984; Featherstone 1987, 1991): 'consumer culture latches onto the prevalent self-preservation conception of the body, which encourages the individual to adopt instrumental strategies to combat deterioration and decay' (Featherstone 1991: 170). In a consumer culture, looking good, feeling good and being healthy become merged as the appearance of the body is seen to reflect the inner self.

Featherstone (1987) argues that consumerism has fundamentally changed the ways that people see themselves and view their bodies. Several features of healthism such as linking youth, beauty and health, a focus on body maintenance and individual responsibility, and anxiety about ageing and death are also features of contemporary consumer culture. For example, individuals are encouraged to monitor their bodies and compare them to those of celebrities or models. Negligence in body maintenance resulting in physical signs of ageing such as grey hair, wrinkles or weight gain 'become interpreted as signs of moral laxitude' (Featherstone 1991: 178). Thus body maintenance is seen as a virtuous activity. Health promotion offers a similar message.

> However much health educationalists appeal to the rationality of self preservation and offer the incentives of longevity and lowered risk of disease, their body maintenance messages are strongly influenced by the consumer culture idealisation of youth and the body beautiful.
>
> (Featherstone 1991: 183)

The emphasis on bodily maintenance and bodily surveillance found in lifestyle-focused health promotion and health education, it is argued, reflects and reproduces the commodification and commercialisation of bodies and health (Featherstone 1987, 1991). In this situation 'there is a commercialisation of health in that people are constructed as health consumers who may consume healthy lifestyles' (Nettleton 1995: 49).

Sociologists writing about lifestyle and consumption also point to widespread adherence to a notion that health can be purchased. Evidence of the belief that health can be purchased through the consumption of healthy lifestyle symbols can be seen in the success of the beauty and fitness industry (Featherstone 1991; Williams 1998). Wearing sunglasses, sports shoes, and clothes with sports brand labels, using organic or 'natural' beauty products, jogging, going to the gym, and practising yoga have all been associated with a healthy lifestyle. The purchasing of such healthful signs is seen as responsible and valuable. In a lifestylist society the body is regarded as a consumer commodity. The desire to be perceived by others as being in good health is necessary for the successful marketing of the body as a commodity. A fit body is seen as a sign of 'competence, self control, and self discipline' (Nettleton 1995: 51).

The major reason why sociologists view the commodification and commercialisation of health and bodies as problematic is that a lifestyle approach implies that not having a healthy lifestyle is a form of weakness or irresponsibility. This ignores the fact that the consumption of a 'healthy' lifestyle, like all forms of consumption, 'is constrained by the social and material contexts in which people live out their lives' (Nettleton 1995: 51). Annandale (1998) describes consumption as a new axis of inequality. She argues that the lifestyles and health practices associated with a lifestyle approach to health are not practically accessible to those at the bottom of the ladder. 'For these people, maintaining health and gaining access to health care is an intractable problem' (Annandale 1998: 121).

A lifestyle approach continues the modernist scientific emphasis of medicine

The argument presented by authors such as Petersen and Lupton (1996) and Hughes (1994) that medical ways of understanding health and illness in terms of lifestyle are a continuation of the medical tradition which deals with such issues in a modernist, science-based manner might at first seem rather strange. Medicine is after all widely accepted as dealing with issues of sickness and health in a modernist and science-based manner (Freund and McGuire 1991). This critique can be understood, however, if two background issues are considered.

First, in medicine explaining disease in terms of lifestyle has been represented as a successful attempt to overcome the reductive nature of traditional medical understandings of disease in favour of a complex biopsychosocial understanding (Launer and Lindsey 1997; Usherwood 1999). Critics such as Hughes (1994) or Petersen and Lupton (1996) argue that an over-reliance on conceptions of risk in epidemiological and public health understandings of lifestyle serves to negate this aim by transforming complex socially and culturally embedded behaviours and practices into quantified risk factors for disease. Such an approach fails to recognise the complexity of the social patterning of illness. Further, the production of risk factors serves to 'sanitise, trivialise and abstract illness and disease into information in a database. The expectation is generated that merely altering a few wrong numbers will enable people to become healthy' (Hughes 1994: 65).

Quantification and abstraction also serve to erase the lived realities of illness and disability. Hughes (1994) argues that reducing illness or health to simplistic measurements contributes to a generalised insensitivity towards those who are ill or even those who are seen to be placing themselves at risk of disease in the future. This abstraction and distancing tend to foster the moralistic judgements and discrimination associated with a lifestyle approach.

Thus, this argument posits that while lifestyle models might seem to be a reflection of a different type of medical explanation for disease, the way that lifestyle arguments are constructed in epidemiology and public health means that they are simply more of the same. That is, lifestyle models are little or no different from more traditional medical explanatory models and carry the same burden of weaknesses.

The second issue underpinning this criticism is more complex. Throughout the second half of the twentieth century, writers from many fields but in particular philosophy and the sociology of science have argued successfully that scientific knowledge should not be viewed as an accurate representation of a natural truth but instead as socially constructed knowledge which reflects historically and culturally specific ideas and assumptions (Hesse 1963; Kuhn 1970; Arney and Bergen 1984; Harding 1991; Webster 1991; Atkinson 1995). From this perspective, all scientific facts are 'products of the scientific communities from which they emerge . . . our presumed stable realities are in fact realised within variable discursive contexts' (Nettleton 1995: 21).

One result of this debate is that medical knowledge and practice have been shown to incorporate considerable sociocultural values (Wright and Treacher 1982a, 1982b; Gordon 1988a): 'What is being proposed is not that medicine is unscientific because it is permeated by social forces: but in contrast, that both medicine and science are inherently social enterprises' (Wright and Treacher 1982b: 7).

Writers have used these arguments to suggest that the modernist and scientific approach is not as it has been represented to be, that is stable, objective and impartial. This critique has frequently been focused on the institution of medicine and the medical management of sickness and health (e.g. Zola 1972; Navarro 1976, 1986; Illich 1979; Kirmayer 1988). In this context, medical claims that lifestyle arguments are valid and useful because they are supported by scientific research and modern methods of population measurement and surveillance are not seen as convincing or desirable (Brandt 1991).

In addition, the critique of science reveals a contradiction within the medical use of lifestyle models. As discussed above, lifestyle arguments rely heavily on cultural knowledges about right and wrong, clean and dirty, healthy and unhealthy. However, the use of statistics, risk factor jargon and the weighty scientific legitimacy of epidemiological research present lifestyle arguments as being ahistorical, objective and rational. Petersen and Lupton in particular express a deep distrust of a lifestyle approach precisely because it is widely represented as a value-free modern scientific solution to the long-established problems of poor health and inequalities in health, when closer analysis shows it to be 'at its core a moral enterprise, in that it involves prescriptions about how we should live our lives' (1996: xii).

Conclusion

Sociology has considerable investment as a discipline in emphasising the importance of social factors to health. If social factors are considered to be a medically legitimate way of understanding health and disease, then sociological theorising and research about these issues increase in value and are likely to attract increased funding. In consequence the overall prestige of sociology is lifted through association (Strong 1984; Brandt 1991).

Furthermore, sociologists have contributed considerably to the development of epidemiological and public health explanations for disease and health that emphasise the role of lifestyle as a determinant. Classical sociology was among the first academic disciplines to demonstrate that health and disease are socially patterned and socially determined (Abel 1991; Cockerham *et al.* 1997). Since the 1970s sociological research and theorising about chronic illness, sexual behaviour, drug use, exercise and leisure, education and health and, later, HIV/AIDS have been used as a basis for many preventive health, health education and health promotion programmes.

However, throughout the 1980s and 1990s medical sociologists became increasingly dissatisfied with the way that their research findings and theories about social factors and health were being interpreted and translated into epidemiological and health promotion lifestyle models. A widely stated sociological criticism is that medical scientists have produced a notion of lifestyle which is overly focused on individual behaviours and attributes and thus divorced from culture and society (e.g. Fitzgerald 1994; Bunton *et al.* 1995). This reductive conception has reduced the ability of epidemiological and public health models of lifestyle, health and disease to adequately account for the social patterning or determining of health and disease. It has also resulted in a medical approach to lifestyle which is a poor orientating framework for disease prevention, as can be seen in the poor outcomes of lifestyle-focused health promotion and health education (Bunton and Macdonald 1992; Charles and Walters 1994; Richmond 1997).

It is not only the reductive aspects of the medical understanding of lifestyle that have attracted sociological critique but also, as pointed out earlier, the cultural aspects: its potential to encourage moralistic and discriminatory views and practices; its capacity to extend medicalisation and medical surveillance; its ability to magnify the concern people have with risk and the accompanying commercialisation of such concern into the sale of body and health products; and, finally, the way in which medical understandings of lifestyle are treated as scientific facts.

This critique has been widely accepted within the sociological literature. It sits easily in the canon of medical sociology/sociology of health and illness which has always had as a basis the critique (either implicit or explicit) of the institution of medicine, medical knowledge and practice (Strong 1984; Turner 1987; Brandt 1991; Pescosolido and Kronenfeld 1995; Grbich 1999). Writers criticising a lifestyle approach as found in epidemiology or sections of public health have generally been better at suggesting that this approach is a flawed explanatory framework than they have been at suggesting an alternative medical framework for explaining the social determinants of health and disease:

> Theirs is the politics of critique; within their hermeneutics of suspicion, anything smelling of prescription is dangerous. The political point seems not so much what we *should* do – that question represents the old medical and public health paradigm – but how we should think and talk about our bodies' health and illness.
>
> (Frank 1997: 104)

Despite this absence of clear directives about how current medical ideas about lifestyle could be changed for the better, there is an implicit claim underlying the critical sociological writings outlined in both this chapter and the previous one that sociologists are far better equipped to explain and address the social determinants of health and disease than are those writing within medicine. The constant comparison made by the sociologists reviewed in this chapter between medical and sociological understandings of lifestyle in which differences between the two are described as problems can be viewed as a disciplinary claim by sociologists. The underlying assumption seems to be that if medicine is to fully explain the social, it needs to become more like sociology. As Strong (1979a) and Williams (2001) argue, medical sociology has a 'vested interest in the diminution of the medical empire as currently constituted' (Williams 2001: 135).

However, criticism of contemporary medical understandings of lifestyle is criticism of the social model of health and illness which social scientists themselves encouraged medicine to adopt in place of the biological reductionism of the medical model. The irony is that when medicine did adopt a social model of health and illness (lifestyle) this did not make medicine more sociological. Instead sociological arguments about the social determinants of health and illness became less sociological and more medical.

A number of authors stress the widespread influence of lifestyle models of disease promoted in the new public health. They are particularly concerned about the supposed dominance of lifestyle models of disease underpinning the new public health because they consider this to be an inherently controlling enterprise concerned with correcting and 'making up' specific types of individuals (Petersen and Lupton 1996: 174):

Lifestyle models do seem to be among the most widely used explanatory frameworks within the field of public health (Richardson 1991; Bunton and Burrows 1995). Whether they have in fact pervaded other medical spheres is harder to ascertain due to a lack of empirical research on this issue. Other than in epidemiology and public health we do not know how doctors construct, interpret and apply ideas about lifestyle to make sense of health, illness and disease. Nor do we know how medical understandings of lifestyle utilise lay understandings of lifestyle.

To address these areas of underdevelopment, medical understandings of lifestyle were examined empirically in a qualitative multimethod study (Morgan 1997). The methods used were a thematic textual review of medical and lay texts, twenty in-depth interviews with doctors, observation of fifty-two doctor/patient consultations with a general practitioner and observation of Emily's own eight doctor/patient consultations. These data were analysed in an iterative process that utilised coding for the purpose of theory generation (Miles and Huberman 1994).

Thematic analysis of formalised written medical and lay accounts of lifestyle was undertaken. These had the advantage of being stable and of being written across a thirty-year time period, thus providing an overview of medical and lay understandings from the 1970s, when the early epidemiological research into the lifestyle basis of cardiovascular disease was first reported, to the late 1990s. This is the thirty-year period in which the contemporary medical understandings of lifestyle, described in chapter 1, have been operating (Crawford 1978, 1980; Armstrong 1979, 1983, 1995; Fitzgerald 1994). The documents examined were medical journals and medical textbooks selected on the recommendation of clinical school librarians and, in the case of textbooks, those cited frequently in journal articles. Public health policy documents of the same time period were also examined, as were contemporary brochures on lifestyle distributed in doctors' surgeries. In addition, lay accounts of lifestyle were sourced from self-help books, complementary medicine texts, popular magazines and pamphlets on alternative therapies, fitness and nutrition (the pamphlets collected from chemists' shops and health food shops).

The interviews provided information about the subjective meanings of lifestyle for doctors and their interpretations of these (Denzin and Lincoln 1994; Rice and Ezzy 1999). They also allowed for comparisons to be made between individual doctors and between different types of doctors. The twenty doctors (ten male, ten female) were deliberately recruited from a range of different medical fields. Twelve were general practitioners, two were medical residents and six were medical specialists (one epidemiologist, two oncologists, one obstetrician, one dermatologist, one haematologist). Most medical work involves decision making and advice giving. It does not involve relatively abstract deliberations on the nature and content of medical knowledge. Talking about lifestyle as a concept that was not necessarily fixed or stable was a new way of thinking for the doctors and many of them were uncomfortable with or unused to talking about their medical knowledge in this way.

To gain an understanding of the way that doctors construct understandings of lifestyle and apply these during medical practice, fifty-two doctor/patient consultations were observed over a period of four days. The purpose of these observations was to explore how a single doctor talked to his patients about lifestyle and to investigate how he applied his understandings of lifestyle during medical practice.

Emily conducted observations during eight of her own consultations, six with a general practitioner, one with a dermatologist and one with a gynaecologist. We chose to include personal observation in the methods used to collect data for two reasons. First, we were committed to making use of as many different types of data as possible to add to the richness and density of our interpretations (Jackson 1989; Clough 1992; Denzin and Lincoln 1994). Second, only through participant observation could Emily include in the analysis the experience of how a patient feels when a doctor talks about lifestyle in certain ways (Blumer 1969; Lofland and Lofland 1984).

Data collection and analysis were performed concurrently and all the various forms of data were analysed using an iterative coding technique. The list of codes arising from this process included the following: uncertainty,

certainty, family, stress, control, cause/causation, action, education, health promotion, relationships, lifestyle, lifestyles, everyday life, normality, smoking, drinking, blame, fate, responsibility, patients, luck, exercise, risk factors, risk, fat, prevention, journals, research, clinical knowledge, expertise, cancer, diabetes, asthma, sexually transmitted infections, cardiovascular diseases, circulatory diseases, health, disease, advice, patients wanting to know why, heredity, individualism, change, own experiences, vulnerability, collecting information, morality, healthy lifestyle, your own lifestyle, their lifestyle, patient's lifestyle, fitness, ageing, doctors' feelings. As interviews progressed and analysis of transcripts continued these codes were grouped into identifiable themes; that is, coded data were transformed into meaningful data (Coffey and Atkinson 1996).

In summary, the research was conducted within an interpretative constructionist paradigm. Medical understandings of lifestyle were explored using four different types of data that provided a range of rich qualitative material. These data were analysed using an iterative technique imbued by grounded theory (Mostyn 1985; Dey 1993; Layder 1993; Strauss and Corbin 1994; Seidman 1998). The result was an understanding of the ways lifestyle is conceptualised in medical and lay texts and how individual medical doctors from different medical fields construct, interpret and apply explanatory models for health, illness and disease that focus on lifestyle. This understanding will be described in the following two chapters.

In the next chapter we examine medical texts and medical journals to understand how lifestyle is conceptualised in written documents in medicine and we compare such conceptualisations with those in non-medical documents. In chapter 5 we look at doctors' understanding of lifestyle as expressed in interviews and as inferred through doctor/patient interactions. We do this by focusing on three questions: How is lifestyle being conceptualised in different medical fields? How do individual doctors understand lifestyle? How do lay and medical conceptions of lifestyle interrelate in medical understandings of lifestyle?

4   Lifestyle in medical
and lay texts

Introduction

This chapter presents the results of the thematic review of medical and lay texts. This review provides an initial exploration of medical understandings of lifestyle guided by the research question: How are medical understandings of lifestyle being constructed in different medical fields?

In response to this question, we demonstrate that different medical fields utilise different understandings of lifestyle: there is no unified medical understanding of what lifestyle is or how this might relate to sickness and health. Rather, there is a range of different conceptions of medicine identifiable within medical texts from different medical fields.

To describe these different medical conceptions of lifestyle a typology is outlined. The typology is not intended to describe all the different ways that medical people could conceptualise lifestyle in relation to sickness and health. What it does provide is additional context and a working terminology that will then be used to refer to different medical conceptions of lifestyle in the next chapter (chapter 5) which explores doctors' understandings of lifestyle.

In addition to medical texts, also reviewed were a number of lay publications that address issues of lifestyle, health and disease, for example women's magazines, alternative health texts and self-help books. The review of lay texts was conducted as an initial response to the research question: How do lay and medical understandings of lifestyle interrelate? This review resulted in the construction of a typology of two lay approaches to explaining health and disease in terms of lifestyle, that were apparent in these texts. As with the typology of medical conceptions of lifestyle, this typology of lay conceptions is not intended to describe all of the different ways that lay people conceptualise lifestyle. It does, however, provide a terminology to refer to two ways that lifestyle is being represented outside medicine. In chapter 5, this terminology is used in conjunction with other sociological research into lay knowledges about lifestyle in order to explore the ways that lay and medical conceptions of lifestyle interrelate in doctors' constructions of lifestyle.

The chapter concludes with a summary of the different medical and lay conceptions of lifestyle identified in the textual review and discusses textual representations of lifestyle in general. Some implications for medical practice of the conceptions of lifestyle identified in medical and lay texts are also raised.

Epidemiological and public health texts

Conceptions of lifestyle vary between the fields of epidemiology and public health. This was discussed in detail in chapter 1, so these differences are only briefly summarised below for the purpose of describing a typology of epidemiological and public health conceptions of lifestyle. However, as variation within each field is not described in chapter 1, this will be discussed in detail after the summary.

Epidemiology is a scientific research discipline seeking to increase knowledge about the causes and distribution of disease. Epidemiological understandings of lifestyle are grounded by the parameters of epidemiological research. They are reductive in that lifestyle is conceptualised in terms of distinct and isolated behaviours and practices which may be risk factors for various diseases. The epidemiological interest in lifestyle is orientated towards the identification of the causes of disease (with cause being understood within a probabilistic conception of causality and risk) in populations and patterns of disease and health in populations (e.g. Last 1988; Shy 1997; Rothman 1998). The following definition of lifestyle, taken from a dictionary of epidemiology, sums up the epidemiological understanding of lifestyle:

> Lifestyle: The set of habits and customs that is influenced, modified, encouraged or constrained by the lifelong process of socialisation. These habits and customs include use of substances such as alcohol, tobacco, coffee, tea, dietary habits, exercise, etc., which have important implications for health and are often the subject of epidemiologic investigation.
>
> (Last 1988: 73)

In contrast, public health is an applied discipline aiming to design, implement and assess strategies to improve health and prevent disease. Unlike epidemiological texts which display an internally consistent and coherent understanding of lifestyle, public health texts reflect two distinct public health discourses, each of which has a distinct conception of lifestyle. These are risk factor health promotion and the new public health.

In risk factor health promotion, conceptions of lifestyle are similar to those found in epidemiology with the important difference that instead of lifestyle risks being expressed in terms of populations they are represented as the property of individuals. In addition, risk factor health promotion is orientated towards education and the modification of lifestyle behaviours and habits rather than the identification of lifestyle risks (as in epidemiology) (e.g. Krug 1995; Stampfer *et al.* 2000).

Conceptions of lifestyle in the discourse of the new public health differ from risk factor health promotion in being strongly influenced by holistic and structural thinking from nursing, sociology and psychology. The result of this is a biopsychosocial conception of *lifestyles*. In this way of conceptualising lifestyle, behaviours and practices considered to influence health or increase risk of disease are located within a wider social context (e.g. World Health Organization 1986; O'Connor and Parker 1995). The focus remains on education and change. However, this is achieved through structural means such as workplace reform rather than through the education of individuals. The differences between epidemiological, risk factor health promotion and new public health conceptions of lifestyle are summarised in Table 4.1.

Like other sociological typologies utilising ideal types, this typology is a useful aid for discussion, critique and comparison. However, it also serves to mask the variation that was apparent within epidemiological and public health texts. This variation is discussed below.

Variation within epidemiological texts

Within epidemiological texts constructions of lifestyle varied. This was evident both when textbooks or journals from different decades were considered and when different types of texts were examined, for example journals and textbooks.

Epidemiological textbooks devote very little space to discussions of lifestyle. Lifestyle is rarely listed in their indexes, and is usually only referred to within the body of the book when examples are being given of risk factors for certain diseases. In the majority of cases these diseases are coronary heart disease and some cancers (e.g. MacMahon and Pugh 1970; Olsen and Trichopoulos 1992; Gordis 1996; Rothman 1998). Thus, while ideas about lifestyle are some of the more prominent epidemiological products in the world outside epidemiology, within epidemiology models of lifestyle and disease are only one of many available explanatory frameworks. The fact that epidemiological textbooks, which as a rule are 'how to do it' texts, make limited mention of lifestyle as a topic is also a reflection of their focus on research methods and statistics (Fleck 1979). When textbooks from different decades were compared (1970s, 1980s and 1990s), lifestyle was rarely in the index or chapter titles of 1970s texts, was mentioned slightly more frequently in 1980s texts and was more common in 1990s texts (e.g. MacMahon and Pugh 1970; Holland 1970; Alderson 1983; Feinstein 1985; Olsen and Trichopoulos 1992; Rothman 1998). In later texts lifestyle was discussed in relation to a number of conditions while in texts from the 1970s and early 1980s it was only discussed in relation to cardiovascular disease.

Table 4.1 Comparison of epidemiological, risk factor health promotion and new public health conceptions of lifestyle

Dimension	Epidemiology	Risk factor health promotion	New public health
Principal concern	Studying the distribution and determinants of health and disease in specified populations	Improving health and reducing disease in populations by producing modifications of behaviours deemed to be risk factors for disease in individuals; health education	Improving health and reducing disease in populations through factors such as healthy public policy, enhancing life skills, health education, preventive medicine and community empowerment
Models of thinking	Medical model of disease/statistical methods of research; understanding disease in terms of populations	Medical model of disease; the application of epidemiological research to inequalities in morbidity and mortality; the 'causes' of disease in terms of individual lifestyle factors and to a lesser extent environmental factors; emphasises individual responsibility	Biopsychosocial model of disease and health; theory and practice of the welfare state, WHO, social sciences and nursing, empowerment, citizenship
Definition of lifestyle	Modifiable social factors (as opposed to biological factors) which have a negative impact on physical health; in the 1970s focus only on cardiovascular disease; by the 1990s a large range of diseases considered in terms of possible lifestyle determinants	Behaviours and attributes of individuals which are deemed to be risk factors for disease; most commonly cardiovascular disease, adult onset diabetes, lung cancer, sexually transmitted infections and stroke	Not limited to factors deemed to be risk factors for disease but also includes a generalised conception of 'styles' of living which impact positively and negatively on physical and emotional health
The social	Understood as behavioural, non-biological	Understood as modifiable behaviours or as the immediate social environment of individuals	Behaviours and attributes embedded in structural, cultural, historical and political situation

Risk	Important to overall conception of lifestyle; mathematical risk, the probability of disease in terms of populations, levels of risk	Primary focus of conception of lifestyle; the property of individuals, all or nothing terms, risk and cause are blurred	Uses both epidemiological and risk factor conceptions of risk but risk is not the primary focus of this conception of lifestyle
Lifestyle as a determinant of disease or lifestyle and the prevention of disease	Determinant of disease	Prevention of disease	Prevention of disease, maintenance and improvement of health

Lifestyle is a more common topic in epidemiological journals than in epidemiological textbooks, for example the *International Journal of Epidemiology, Epidemiology and Society* and the *American Journal of Epidemiology*. Lifestyle factors are often the focus of epidemiological research seeking to identify the causes or risks at, or the prognosis after diagnosis for, conditions such as heart disease, infertility, some cancers, social inequalities in health and viral diseases such as hepatitis and, during the 1980s/early 1990s, HIV/AIDS. Thus articles which publish research results frequently refer to lifestyle (e.g. Chang-Claude and Frentzel-Beyme 1993; Huang *et al.* 1996; Twisk *et al.* 1997).

References to lifestyle have increased in epidemiological journal articles, becoming more common through the 1970s, 1980s and 1990s. Furthermore, an examination of journal articles over this period shows that the lifestyle framework has been expanded from the 1970s focus which was almost exclusively on cardiovascular disease to include additional diseases such as asthma, diabetes, sexually transmitted infections, cataracts and arthritis (Terris 1987).

In addition to this extension of the lifestyle framework beyond cardiovascular disease, journal articles also demonstrate that epidemiological arguments about how lifestyle might be a disease determinant have become increasingly sophisticated over time. For example, epidemiological research into lifestyle and coronary heart disease in the 1960s and 1970s established relationships between diets high in animal fats, low exercise levels and smoking and the development of coronary artery disease (Australian Institute of Health and Welfare 1998). In the 1980s this was refined and the importance of cholesterol was highlighted. However, further research in the late 1980s and 1990s has shown the relationship between diet, exercise and cholesterol levels to be much smaller than originally supposed, and genetic and bacterial aspects of arterial disease are now highlighted. In addition, cholesterol levels are now recognised as only one of the important aspects of blood lipids and a range of different fats are now recognised as part of the multicasual pathway to artery disease (Hulley *et al.* 1992; Oliver 1992; Kleiner 1995).

> Our knowledge is still largely incomplete regarding the relationship between dietary factors and the major diseases of our culture. These illnesses include not only cancer and heart disease, which have received the most attention, but also congenital malformations, degenerative conditions of the eye, fractures, and many infectious diseases that are hypothesised to be influenced by the nutritional status of the host.
>
> (Willett 1990: 17)

Variation within public health texts

As with epidemiological texts, there are variations in the ways that lifestyle is represented between and within different public health texts and between texts published in different decades. Differences between texts are often reflections of the different public health discourses discussed in detail in chapter 1 and summarised briefly above. These different public health discourses of lifestyle frequently coexist within the same text and boundaries between them are often indistinct. There was also variation in the ways that lifestyle was conceptualised between textbooks and journal articles.

For example, articles in the *Australian and New Zealand Journal of Public Health*, the *British Journal of Public Health and Medicine*, the *Journal of Health Education*, and *Health Promotion Journal of Australia* were usually either examples of epidemiological research being published in public health journals or were discussions and evaluations of various health promotion programmes based on risk factor health promotion. As such, they often reflected epidemiological and risk factor health promotion constructions of lifestyle situated within a biomedical framework of disease. It is not surprising that public health journals would favour epidemiological research. Scientific journals have a specific role in formalised scientific knowledge, which is to publish up-to-date research findings using esoteric language for an expert audience.

In contrast, policy documents such as *Better Health for All by the Year 2000* (Australian Institute for Health and Welfare 1998), the *Alma Ata Declaration* (World Health Organization 1978) or the *Ottawa Charter* (World Health Organization 1986) usually reflect a broader biopsychosocial view of lifestyle situated within a notion of health conceptualised not in biomedical terms, such as the absence of disease or infirmity, but as a state of complete physical, mental and social wellbeing understood as a fundamental human right (World Health Organization 1986). For example, in the *Adelaide Recommendations* – which were the result of the second international conference on health promotion, building on the *Ottawa Charter* (World Health Organization 1986) – the main aim of healthy public policy is described as creating a 'supportive environment to enable people to lead healthy lives. Such policy makes healthy choices possible or easier for citizens. It makes social and physical environments health-enhancing' (Adelaide Conference 1988: 2). As an indication of the way that traditional lifestyle concerns are situated in a wider framework, the key areas identified as immediate priorities in the development of health public policy were supporting the health of women, food and nutrition, tobacco and alcohol and creating supportive environments (Adelaide Conference 1988).

Public health textbooks vary in their representations of lifestyle. The breadth of these texts means that examples of both the public health discourses on lifestyle and epidemiological constructions of lifestyle, health and disease are found within the same book. Textbooks published since the mid-1980s generally advocate a new public health approach, thus utilising those conceptions of lifestyle. However, discussions of epidemiological data and existing health promotion programmes within those same books frequently utilised a risk factor health promotion conception of lifestyle (e.g. Badura and Kickbusch 1991; Lawson 1991). This is a reflection of the difference between public health theory and policy and the actual implementation of public health programmes. While the aims and theory of the new public health are very broad, the implementation of such policies has generally been restrictive. Richmond (1997) argues that this has been the case in most western countries because the structural, cultural and environmental level of change advocated in the new public health is difficult, expensive and slow. Implementation of such a broad-scale agenda would also challenge entrenched institutions and ideologies already present in the health care sector. These include managerialism (economic rationalism), the medical profession (also medically allied groups such as physiotherapists, psychologists, etc.) and powerful groups such as the tobacco lobby (Richmond 1997).

Health promotion material such as the leaflets and posters found in doctors' surgeries differed from journal articles, textbooks and policy documents. While these leaflets and posters usually reflected a risk factor health promotion view of lifestyle, it was a particularly reductive one. These texts also utilised a highly personalised approach to lifestyle. Phrases such as 'your lifestyle' were common. This is quite different from other types of public health texts that are written not for the people whose lifestyles are under discussion but for the policy makers, doctors, nurses and dieticians who are trying to change and modify *other people's* lifestyles.

An interesting feature of these texts is the tension within health promotion publications published by pharmaceutical companies or industry boards. These have to advocate medically acceptable lifestyle advice in order to be distributed in medical settings, while at the same time encouraging the consumption of certain goods for the sake of profit. For example, the Australian Dairy Corporation publishes a range of pamphlets advising people to include more calcium in their diet and the Australian Meat Marketing Board publishes a range of pamphlets advising people of the importance of iron in the diet.

In the case of pharmaceutical companies, lifestyle advice is treated in the way that doctors often treat alternative medicine, that is as 'complementary medicine'. For example, in a pamphlet published by Pfizer titled *If you have high blood pressure . . .*, the first two sections explain what high blood pressure is and that it should be treated 'by your doctor using appropriate medication'. The next section, titled 'What you should do to help yourself', describes how many individuals are able to treat their high blood pressure through lifestyle modification. However, the final sections advise that high blood pressure is very dangerous and suggest that lifestyle changes should be used in conjunction with supervised medical treatment using pharmaceutical drugs.

Public health texts of all kinds, technical and lay, are thus unclear on the meaning of the term lifestyle. As a *term*, lifestyle is often used to refer to both specific risk factors and non-specified social factors. In the latter case, specific risk factors for disease are addressed separately (e.g. smoking, blood lipids, body mass index (BMI), unsafe sex) while the term lifestyle is used to refer to other unspecified non-biological factors. In this context, lifestyle is frequently used to talk about exercise, e.g. the phrases 'sedentary lifestyle' or simply 'unhealthy lifestyles'.

'Mainstream' medical texts

This section describes the ways that lifestyle is conceptualised in 'mainstream' medical journals, general practice texts and undergraduate textbooks, using texts from the bachelor of medicine degree at the University of Tasmania. Conceptions of lifestyle from medical fields other than epidemiology or public health are of particular interest for two reasons. The first is that previous sociological writing has not addressed the ways that lifestyle might be conceptualised in medical fields other than epidemiology or public health. Second, the majority of doctors interviewed or observed in this research were general practitioners or hospital specialists. Both of these types of doctors are unlikely to read specialist epidemiological or public health texts but are likely to read mainstream medical journals and general practice texts, and, in the case of the young doctors and the doctors who lecture at the medical school, to have some level of familiarity with current undergraduate medical textbooks. Thus their individual understandings of lifestyle (which will be explored in chapter 5) are likely to be imbued with the various conceptions of lifestyle found in mainstream medical texts. Thus the terminology to refer to these will be very useful.

Furthermore, as argued in chapter 2, medical understandings of lifestyle may well transcend the preventive focus of public health (and to a lesser extent epidemiology) because prevention takes up only a small proportion of everyday clinical practice. Thus if doctors are constructing understandings of lifestyle to serve as explanatory frameworks for disease (or health), then they may be using lifestyle in different ways to those commonly found in epidemiology or public health. This review of mainstream medical texts serves as an initial investigation of the question: Do conceptions of lifestyle in medical fields other than epidemiology and public health transcend the preventive focus found in those two fields?

The textual review demonstrates that the most common conceptualisation of lifestyle in mainstream medical texts is one informed by the epidemiological notion of lifestyle factors as risk factors for certain diseases. In mainstream medical texts, lifestyle is represented as a risk factor for coronary heart disease, sexually transmitted disease and some cancers (e.g. McWhinney 1989; Cormack *et al.* 1992). However, rather than being a direct reflection of epidemiology, mainstream medical conceptions of lifestyle were also very similar to those found in risk factor health promotion.

Unlike published epidemiological research about lifestyle (which was generally concerned with lifestyle as a determinant of disease), research about lifestyle published in the mainstream medical journals was much less likely to ask about determinants of disease and more likely to be concerned with either patient knowledge about lifestyle factors or the impact of various types of intervention on morbidity or mortality, for example lifestyle change and cardiovascular disease (e.g. Oldenburg *et al.* 1992), trials of diet modification for lowering plasma cholesterol levels (Johnston *et al.* 1995) or the end results of stress management courses. This is compatible with the clinical focus of mainstream medical texts. It is also closely aligned with a risk factor health promotion approach to lifestyle.

Second, unlike epidemiology and, again, more like risk factor health promotion, mainstream medical conceptions of lifestyle factors are individualised and personalised. In this context the doctors authoring these texts describe patients' lifestyles as putting them at risk of developing certain diseases (e.g. Gammon 1990; Murtagh 1994). Mainstream medical texts do, however, demonstrate a significant difference between a public health and mainstream medical approach to risk factor intervention. In public health texts, while actual programmes are individually targeted, the underlying aim is to achieve a small modification in lifestyle practices across the population in order to lower the risk profile for the population (Wilkinson 1996). In mainstream medical texts, however (probably because such texts have a clinical focus which is by its nature individualist), a more common approach is to advise that patients whose lifestyle behaviours place them at highest risk of developing disease be targeted individually and their own risk profile lowered (Pearson 1989; Ashenden *et al.* 1998).

An example of this is the practice of lifestyle counselling by doctors. In lifestyle counselling doctors (usually general practitioners) are expected to identify their patients' 'unhealthy' or 'risky' lifestyle practices and advise them to change these with the aim of reducing their risk of disease (e.g. Nutting 1986; Stott 1986; RACGP 1998). The most common lifestyle issues which doctors are advised to target are smoking, alcohol consumption, dietary behaviour and exercise (Ashenden *et al.* 1998). While studies of the effectiveness of lifestyle counselling by doctors (measured in terms of patients who change these behaviours) suggest that even when patients do make recommended lifestyle changes these are rarely maintained in the long term, medical texts still strongly advise doctors to offer lifestyle counselling (Yeager *et al.* 1996; Ashenden at al. 1998). For example, the United States National Institute of Health recommends

> the development of programs for health professionals to communicate to patients the importance of regular physical activity. .... It is highly probable that people will be more likely to increase their physical activity if their health care professional counsels them to do so.
>
> (NIH 1996: 244–5)

A further way that risk factors are personalised in medical texts is when they are discussed in relation to diagnosis (e.g. Furner and Ross 1993; Wodak 1993). In a textbook teaching clinical methods for general practitioners a selection of annotated transcripts from medical consultations are presented together with commentary and discussion about how most effectively to manage general practice consultations (Gammon 1990). Lifestyle information about diet, physical activity, smoking and alcohol consumption are listed by Gammon (1990) as issues to be considered by general practitioners as part of the diagnostic process.

The differences between epidemiological, risk factor health promotion and mainstream medical conceptions of lifestyle risk are summarised in Table 4.2.

The tone used in mainstream medical texts discussing lifestyle advice and collecting lifestyle information was paternalistic (e.g. Balint 1964; Balint *et al.* 1970; Hodgkin 1978; Livesey 1986). It was implied that doctors automatically know what is the best lifestyle for a particular patient. It is also strongly implied in these texts that patients cannot be trusted to tell the truth about their own lifestyle. For example, when consultation transcripts are included in the texts (e.g. Gammon 1990) the patients' own comments about their lifestyle are described as examples of stubbornness, ignorance or simply misinformation and never as a reflection of a valid point of view. For example, 'In history taking the attitude should be never to believe what the patient tells and never to disbelieve it; instead search should be made for some other evidence to confirm or refute it' (Gammon 1990: 6).

This attitude, that patients are unable to understand medical information about lifestyle, is not supported by sociological research (Siegler 1981; Buetow 1995; Johanson *et al.* 1998). Such research has demonstrated that patients bring their own types of expert knowledge to the consultation and that they are able to make use of medical ideas about lifestyle in a competent and skilled way.

Table 4.2 Main features of the conceptions of lifestyle risk in mainstream medical texts in comparison with epidemiological or risk factor health promotion

Dimension	Epidemiology	Risk factor health promotion	Mainstream medical
Principal concern	The identification of risk factors and studying the distribution of risk factors in specified populations	Shifting population risk profiles through individually targeted health promotion campaigns aiming to achieve a small modification in lifestyle practices across the population	Improving patient knowledge about lifestyle risk factors, assessing the impact of lifestyle intervention, lifestyle risk as a diagnostic tool
Models of thinking	Medical model of disease, statistical research, population health	Medical model of disease, epidemiology	Medical model of disease, clinical practice
Definition of lifestyle risk	Modifiable social (non-biological) factors which have a negative impact on physical health	Behaviours and attributes of individuals which place them at 'risk' of disease/which 'cause' disease	Behaviours and attributes of individuals which place them at 'risk' of disease/which 'cause' disease
Focus	Population	High-risk populations, targeting individuals	Patients, individuals, 'high-risk individuals'
Application	Research	Health education	Identifying 'at risk' patients, 'lifestyle counselling' preventive medicine
Tone	Impersonal, scientific	Prescriptive, authoritative	Paternalistic, prescriptive, advice giving

In addition to conceptualising lifestyle in terms of risks, several general practice texts also mentioned lifestyle in the context of discussions about undefined 'social factors' impacting on physical health (e.g. McWhinney 1989; Gammon 1990; Morrell 1991; Cormack *et al.* 1992):

> [T]he social diagnosis is always important . . . how will this illness affect and be affected by the patient's work, family or leisure pursuits? . . . When it [the social diagnosis] remains in the background and appears to be of little importance, probably the reason is that the patient's relationships are functioning well. However, if the illness puts undue stress

on the social relationships, they may quickly come to the fore. The doctor needs to be aware that denial of severe family difficulty is very common.

(Gammon 1990: 8)

As can be seen in this quotation, the mainstream medical understanding of the social is focused on the individual and the family rather than on the structural, cultural or environmental as in the new public health. For example, the following quote from a university course guide summarises this approach:

Unit: Community Health (General Practice): Teaches students, in the context of general practice, to recognise and understand commonly met symptoms, diseases, chronic illnesses, and conditions which may endanger life or have serious consequences; the opportunities, methods and limitations of prevention, early diagnosis, and management; the social, cultural ·and environmental circumstances of individuals and families and how these may affect their health; peer based and individual professional competency reviews; the Australian health system, community rural and urban health care resources and services to other disadvantaged groups; and the GP's role as a provider of continuing 'whole person' care.

(University of Tasmania 1999: 486)

However, in addition to the individualist focus found in many mainstream medical texts, several general practice textbooks utilised a broader biopsychosocial definition of lifestyle (e.g. Usherwood 1999). When lifestyle was being conceptualised in a biopsychosocial way, the focus was on patients' psychological states and their immediate social environments (e.g. Livesey 1986; Neighbour 1987; Morrell 1991). Usherwood (1999: 84) argues that family doctors 'have a responsibility which extends beyond the prevention and treatment of physical disease to include emotional and psychosocial issues'. Such a conceptualisation of lifestyle was common in mainstream medical texts that were advocating the desirability of health promotion (defined in terms of enabling all people to increase control over and improve their health) (e.g. RACGP 1998; Rogers *et al.* 1999).

Discussions of lifestyle in these contexts demonstrated an expanded conception of the pathogenic sphere, as discussed in chapter 2 (Lowenberg and Davis 1994). For example, in a report on linking general practice with population health, the authors advise their readers that in contrast to preventive medicine, in health promotion doctors should be concerned with the population as a whole and not just people at risk of specific diseases. They argue that a concern with the everyday life of populations is the difference between a health promotion perspective and a medical approach to disease prevention (Rogers *et al.* 1999).

In addition to the biopsychosocial approach found in mainstream medical texts interested in health promotion, a looser and more ambiguous conception of lifestyle(s) is apparent where the term is used to refer to often unspecified social factors which might be impacting on a patient's health state or to any social factors which seem to be impacted upon by a patient's health state: for example, when an illness or medication is described as impacting on a patient's lifestyle (e.g. Polglase *et al.* 1984) or when a patient's lifestyle is described as contributing to a difficult-to-define non-somatic situation such as suicide (e.g. Schlicht *et al.* 1990) or non-compliance to a medical regime. This conceptualisation of lifestyle was common when lifestyle(s) was being discussed as a management issue for doctors and their patients (e.g. Jackson 1992; Simpson 1993). As in the example discussed earlier of lifestyle being used in diagnosis, when lifestyle is conceptualised in terms of management the preventive focus of epidemiology and public health is widened. The following abstract from an article about managing epilepsy written by two doctors working at the epilepsy unit at Westmead Hospital, Sydney, demonstrates this generalised understanding of lifestyle:

Abstract: OBJECTIVES: To study delay in diagnosis, seizure control, seizure provoking factors, suitable medications and drug side effects in patients with juvenile myoclonic epilepsy. DESIGN: Telephone and personal interview of patients and review of their clinical notes. PARTICI-PANTS AND SETTING: Thirty-six patients attending an epilepsy clinic at a tertiary referral hospital. RESULTS: There was a substantial delay in the diagnosis of juvenile myoclonic epilepsy because the symptom of early morning myoclonus was not specifically sought. Sodium valproate is the drug of choice producing absolute seizure control in 63% of cases (19/30). *Most patients with poor seizure control had provoked seizures only, emphasising the importance of lifestyle in management.*
(Sharpe and Buchanan 1995: 133; italics added)

What can be seen in this conception of lifestyle is an approach informed not by public health or epidemiology but, instead, by conceptions of lifestyle similar to those found in social work, and the sociological chronic illness literature (e.g. Charmaz 1987; Robinson 1993; Thorne 1993). In the chronic illness literature and the social work literature discussions of lifestyle and health focus on how individuals and their families are able to cope successfully with the many demands of chronic illnesses such as asthma, arthritis, diabetes, multiple sclerosis or epilepsy (Knafl and Deatrick 1986; Charmaz 1990; Altschuler 1997).

Coping successfully is usually defined as effective management of the illness so that individuals are able to maintain their 'normal' lifestyle or to develop a lifestyle that is achievable within the limitations imposed by medical treatment and physical capacity. These understandings of lifestyle are permeated by the sociological concepts of normalisation and management.

Normalisation refers to a process whereby individuals and families living with a chronic illness come to define their ill member and their family life as normal: 'Numerous researchers have found that the preferred story for many individuals and families managing a chronic condition is one of normalisation, that is essentially normal persons living normal lives' (Robinson 1993: 9). Management is defined as an active process of applying specific measures to deal with illness concerns (Brooks and Matson 1987). Understanding illness in terms of management highlights the continuous efforts involved in living with a chronic illness.

The implications of this for medical understandings are that a healthy lifestyle is understood in terms not of risk factors for disease but of what is considered normal and desirable by patients, their family and to a lesser extent doctors and other health workers. Disease, illness and medical treatment are all seen as factors which impact (usually negatively) on an individual's attempts to live a normal lifestyle. A lifestyle is viewed as being made up of ordinary tasks and actions such as work, leisure and housework which shifts and changes in response to external pressures (e.g. Gerson *et al.* 1993).

As can be seen from this discussion, mainstream medical constructions of lifestyle, health and disease are interesting because they are so varied. Mainstream medical texts such as journals, general practice texts and undergraduate medical texts demonstrate that outside the fields of epidemiology and public health medical conceptions of lifestyle are diverse and complex. These texts display epidemiological, risk factor health promotion and new public health understandings of lifestyle. They also show variations of these because unlike the research field of epidemiology or public health, both of which are primarily concerned with patterns of disease and disease prevention in populations, mainstream medicine deals with diagnosis and the management of illness conditions in individuals.

In this context structural issues are individualised to focus on the family rather than on wider issues such as unemployment or unsafe working conditions for certain types of workers. The psychological aspect of a biopsychosocial model of lifestyle is emphasised, particularly in relation to lifestyle issues such as family and personal relationships.

In addition, mainstream medical conceptions include characterisations of lifestyle not found in epidemiology or public health. See Table 4.3 for a summary of the distinctive mainstream medical conceptions of lifestyle.

An example of the distinctive nature of medical conceptions of lifestyle identified in general practice texts is the representation of lifestyle issues as pertaining to the present situation rather than the prevention of future situations. Furthermore, lifestyle is often written about in terms of diagnosis, management and treatment for illness [conditions] rather than as risks for disease (Furner and Ross 1993). General practice texts also include broad, 'sweeping notions of 'normal lifestyle' and 'everyday lifestyle'. Here, lifestyle is being considered not in terms of risk but, quite differently, in terms of

Table 4.3 Lifestyle in terms of diagnosis and management, distinctive mainstream medical conceptions of lifestyle

Dimension	Diagnosis	Management
Principal concern	Using knowledge about lifestyle risks as tool for diagnosis; types of people identified in health promotion as being 'at risk' for certain diseases	Managing chronic illness and the treatment of disease, achieving a 'normal' lifestyle
Models of thinking	Clinical models for diagnosis, medical model	Biopsychosocial and medical models, sociological, behavioural and nursing models
Definition of lifestyle	Behaviours or attributes of individuals which are deemed to be risk factors for disease	Styles of living, everyday life
The social	Not applicable, individualist focus	The social lives of the individual whose illness is being managed, particularly their family, personal relationships and work
Risk	Important but blurred with cause	Risk is not a focus

how people want their lives to be, or as something that illness or treatment impact upon (or which might impact on the efficacy of a particular treatment regime).

Variation within mainstream medical texts

As in epidemiological and public health texts, conceptions of lifestyle vary between different mainstream medical texts and within individual texts. Conceptions of lifestyle have also changed over time. This is demonstrated when texts published in different decades are compared (Hasler and Schofield 1984; Usherwood 1999).

Mainstream medical texts such as general practice guides and textbooks, books about primary health care, and journal articles about prevention and family medicine all contain frequent references to lifestyle. As described earlier in this section, these types of texts utilise a range of different conceptions of lifestyle including epidemiological, risk factor health promotion, lifestyle as a diagnostic tool, lifestyle as everyday life which is impacted upon by illness or treatment, and other biopsychosocial conceptions of lifestyle (e.g. Usherwood 1990, 1999; Walsh and McPhee 1992; Cohen *et al.* 1994; Jaen *et al.* 1994).

In contrast to this, medical textbooks from the bachelor of medicine degree at the University of Tasmania do not reflect a concern with lifestyle. Instead, these undergraduate medical textbooks are primarily concerned with scientific medicine (anatomy, physiology, biochemistry) (e.g. Talley and O'Connor 1996; Wilson and Braunwald 1997). This is a reflection of the course material of this undergraduate medical degree which (like other undergraduate medical degrees) is largely focused on biological disorders (and the application of the medical model).

Lifestyle was only touched upon in textbooks for community health, general practice, rural health and to a lesser extent epidemiology and bio-statistics (e.g. Neighbour 1987; Murtagh 1994). These texts provide an individually focused understanding of lifestyle and health. When the term lifestyle is used it is in the context of a brief summary of cardiac risk factors, or of risk factor prevention strategies, or in the context of referring to a patient's wider social environment. When disease or health is mentioned in terms of social settings or characteristics the individual is central to the discussion in the social setting of the family. The structural understanding of lifestyle and health found in sociology and traditional public health is represented in only one recommended textbook for the first year of the degree (Davis and George 1990).

In contrast to undergraduate medical textbooks, mainstream medical journals contain many references to lifestyle although the topic only features in mainstream (non-epidemiological, non-public health and non-specialist) medical journals since the mid-1970s. Lifestyle did not appear as a medical subject heading in these journals before 1971. This is a reflection of the relatively recent nature of epidemiological and public health concern with non-infectious diseases (Terris 1987) and of the expansion of epidemiological ideas and research about lifestyle into other medical fields and popular consciousness which occurred throughout the 1970s (Crawford 1984; Fitzgerald 1994; Petersen and Lupton 1996).

A review of articles from the *Medical Journal of Australia, Modern Medicine Australia, Australian and New Zealand Journal of Medicine* and *Australian Family Physician* found that the number of articles with lifestyle as a key subject heading had increased from nine in the period 1971–6 to forty in the period 1981–6. The number of articles with lifestyle as a key word decreased in the period 1987–90 and then started to increase again 1991–6. The increase from the 1970s and the sharp peak in the early to mid-1980s represented mainly articles about cardiac risk factors. The second climb in the 1990s was partially attributable to articles about risk factors for HIV/AIDS and also to a broadening of the scope of articles where lifestyle was a key subject heading. This reflects the extension of a lifestyle and risk focus to diseases other than cardiac disease.

Articles with lifestyle as a key subject heading were common in the *Medical Journal of Australia* and *Australian Family Physician* and uncommon in the *Australian and New Zealand Journal of Medicine*. *Modern Medicine Australia* had no articles with lifestyle as a key subject heading. The popularity of epidemiological style research in the *Medical Journal of Australia* and the popularity of articles about challenges for medical practice such as illness management and patient care in the *Australian Family Physician* explain this pattern.

Lay texts

As discussed in chapter 1, lay perceptions of lifestyle in relation to health and disease have been the focus of considerable sociological research (e.g. Blaxter 1983, 1990, 1997; Whittaker 1995; Kavanagh and Broom 1998; Wiles 1998). This published research has used interview and survey data to demonstrate the considerable variety that exists within lay perceptions of lifestyle.

In order to establish a working terminology of some prominent lay representations of lifestyle operating within Australian popular culture in the mid- to late- 1990s Emily reviewed a range of lay texts including self-help books, women's magazines, newspapers and alternative medical texts. This review does not reflect the full range of different lay views on lifestyle and health. For example, religious discourses on lifestyle, health and disease are not dealt with in detail. The small info-magazines produced by the Seventh Day Adventist Church and Jehovah's Witnesses contain very similar ideas about lifestyle to those identified in health promotion texts and the self-help and fitness industry except that an emphasis on financial profit is replaced with an emphasis on religious credit. A healthy lifestyle is presented as a vital part of being a Seventh Day Adventist or a Jehovah's Witness. Despite its limited range, the review has allowed for two ideal types of lay conceptions of lifestyle to be added to the typology of medical conceptions presented earlier.

In addition to risk factor health promotion which frequently crosses between lay and medical texts, two additional distinctive approaches to lifestyle and health occurred frequently in the lay texts reviewed. The first of these was common in popular magazines, self-help books, diet and exercise magazines (and also on infotainment television) and we have termed this conception of lifestyle 'self-help, health, beauty and fitness industry'. This way of conceiving lifestyle presents a 'healthy' lifestyle as a marketable commodity. The second lay conception of lifestyle was (as would be expected) dominant in alternative/holistic medical texts but was also common in women's magazines, some self-help books and diet/exercise magazines. This we have called 'alternative/holistic medicine'. See Table 4.4 for a summary of these two lay approaches.

Self-help, health, beauty and fitness industry

Ideas about lifestyle and health in this industry are explicitly centred on the selling of 'lifestyle' information to make monetary profit. Examples include health promotion advertising sponsored by industry bodies such as the Australian Dairy Corporation and the Australian Meat Marketing Board,

Table 4.4 Comparing 'self-help, health, beauty and fitness industry' approach to lifestyle with a 'holistic/alternative medicine' approach

Dimension	Self-help, health, beauty and fitness industry	Holistic/alternative medicine
Principal concern	'Selling' lifestyle 'facts' lifestyle and identity health, youth, beauty, sexual desirability	Promoting wellbeing, preventing disease, advocating a 'healthy lifestyle'.
Models of thinking	Risk factor health promotion, marketing, consumption, individual responsibility	Non-western models of disease, alternative and holistic models of health and disease, occasionally draws on science for legitimacy, individual responsibility
Definition of lifestyle	Something which an individual has, a 'healthy' lifestyle or an 'unhealthy lifestyle' constituted through consumption	All aspects of being, includes physical, spiritual and emotional
Risk	Risk factors as direct causes, individualised, personalised	Rarely mentioned
The social	Individualised	Individualised

the new breed of infotainment television shows such as *Healthy Wealthy and Wise* and *Good Medicine*, books about lifestyle and health written by medical doctors such as *The LS Factor: Lifestyle and Health* by Hetzel and McMichael (1987), health and beauty pages in magazines such as *Cleo* and the *Australian Women's Weekly* and popular magazines which focus explicitly on lifestyle and health such as *Men's Health, Health and Fitness* and *Women and Health*.

In this version of a lifestyle approach, health is a state that is achieved by living a 'healthy lifestyle'. Health can be recognised by a suitably slim and youthful appearance. In the representations of a lifestyle approach to understanding disease found in self-help, fitness, beauty and health texts, health is articulated in terms of an individual's identity as constructed through consumption practices. Individuals, as consumers, are purchasing the signs of a healthy lifestyle (healthy food, exercise clothing and equipment) for their meaning rather than their utility or exchange value (Featherstone 1991; Bauman 1992; Crook *et al.* 1992). This linking of lifestyle, identity and consumption is overt in the cultural products from the self-help, fitness and beauty industry where the body is viewed as a source of investment. Fitness and health are commodities which can be stored as cultural assets (Schilling 1991; Savage *et al.* 1992; Synott 1992; Harvey 1998).

In a time when awareness of the potential health risks of almost any action is heightened and fear of inevitable ageing and death is widespread, the purchasing of health foods, self-help books or videos, exercise clothing and equipment is critical to the formation of a self identity as a healthy person (Warde 1994). It also serves to alleviate feelings of anxiety or guilt about having an unhealthy lifestyle.

This set of ideas about lifestyle and health is strongly informed by risk factor health promotion (thus also by epidemiological research into the determinants of disease). Like risk factor health promotion, information about lifestyle and health/disease is generally presented as medical facts which can be used by the reader as a guide for the ongoing challenge of achieving and maintaining a healthy lifestyle and preventing disease/ disability (e.g. Hetzel and McMichael 1987; Kowalski 1989; Connor and Connor 1991).

As in risk factor health promotion, in self-help, beauty, health and fitness industry conceptions, lifestyle information is frequently discussed in terms of risk. However, representations of lifestyle risk in self-help/fitness and beauty industry texts are even more reductive than those found in risk factor health promotion. In self-help industry texts statements about risk, disease determinants and lifestyle are presented without any of the qualifying statements found in medical texts. Lay readers are not presented with any competing ideas or evidence about lifestyle and health, nor are they provided with any information about how such research results were obtained. Any awareness of differing levels of risk is lost. Risk factors become direct causes as in the following quotation:

> There is a growing recognition that the major causes of disease and disability in contemporary, affluent, Western society are the result of individual behaviours in daily life and that the key to good health lies much more with the prevention than with the cure.
>
> (Hetzel and McMichael 1987: 2)

To a lesser extent, the self-help and fitness industry understandings about lifestyle and health also contain influences from the wellness movement (and other associated sets of ideas about health) in that they refer to 'feeling better' and 'improved self-esteem through fitness', and contain words such as 'vitality', 'energy' and 'wellbeing'. In many cases statements about the 'other' benefits of a healthy lifestyle (other than slimness, youth or disease prevention) are fairly cursory and often appear to be an attempt to provide additional motivation to the reader, especially the type based on immediate gratification. This is demonstrated in the following quote from *Cosmopolitan Magazine*: 'an exercise program will have immediate benefits such as increased feelings of wellbeing and vitality long before weight loss and cardiovascular fitness results become noticeable' (January 1999: 45).

An interesting variation within the self-help/fitness and beauty industry representations of lifestyle is that found in advertising material for miracle cures. These brochures, leaflets and advertisements at the back of some magazines promote books, videos or cassettes which are said to contain information about 'super foods' that prevent and reverse ageing or 'quick and easy' exercise to improve your appearance. Sometimes written by doctors or by skilled lay people with some claim to specialist knowledge, these texts present a lifestyle approach which aims to replace traditional medical therapies such as drugs and surgery and which claims to produce cures in chronic patients.

Another feature of self-help/fitness and beauty industry representations of lifestyle and health is that these frequently utilise ideas and phrases from alternative medicine. It is in fact very difficult to differentiate between alternative/holistic understandings about health and lifestyle and self-help/fitness and beauty industry understandings in many popular texts (Goldstein 2000). Alternative health information is marketable and fashionable (Easthope 1993; Siahpush 1998) and provides far more scope for the authors of self-help texts than the rather limited range of risk factor health promotion.

Alternative/holistic medicine

Holistic and alternative medicine are influential lay discourses on health, bodies and illness (Siahpush 1998). Alternative medicine has risen in popularity since the 1970s. Explanations for this include the women's health movement and gay rights movement, both of which have resulted in opposition towards orthodox medicine, and widespread societal changes in levels of trust accorded to orthodox professionals and expert systems. Siahpush (1998) suggests that the popularity of alternative health is a reflection of postmodern values while Coward stresses the development of new attitudes towards bodies and health:

> The notion of being alternative is considerably more than just doing it differently from orthodox medicine. It is also a symbolic activity. It is a profound expression of a new consciousness which individuals have about health and the body. This involves a commitment to finding a new lifestyle, to pursuing a new well-being, and to finding 'natural' ways of achieving this well-being. Above all it is a new consciousness of the importance of the individual in achieving health.
>
> (1989: 11).

Proponents of alternative health often use the term lifestyle when referring to all aspects of an individual's being, all of which are assumed to affect physical, emotional and spiritual health (e.g. Chopra 1998). In addition to the issues mentioned in other lifestyle theories such as diet, exercise and stress, these also include spiritual, emotional and environmental issues, as illustrated in the following excerpt from an alternative health text:

The reasons for poor health are at least threefold. Firstly there are the obvious physical causes such as an insect sting, a sports injury, a burn or food poisoning. Second there are the circumstances in which we live, including damp or noisy housing, exposure to high levels of radiation and other pollutants and poor working conditions such as sub-standard lighting and seating which will result in postural misalignment. Thirdly, and in my view probably the most important of all, is the emotional component. Grief, shock, anger, frustration and other negative emotions can be just as potent a cause of disease as any physical factor. So by launching into the reasons why eating properly is the indispensable foundation of all good health I am not implying that nothing else matters. We need clean air and sunshine as well as the plants on which we are so dependent. In common with other animals we need regular exercise and because our minds are indelibly linked to our bodies we also have deep spiritual and psychological needs. If these are not met, eventually our bodies will show the symptoms of dis-ease.

(Campion 1996: 10)

Alternative/holistic conceptions of lifestyle are not based around epidemiological notions about statistical relationships between lifestyle factors and the possibility of developing disease. Rather, they are based around the encompassing ideals of holism, new age philosophy and the specific conceptions of the body and disease found in approaches as varied as naturopathy, reiki, acupuncture, shiatsu, eastern mysticism, paganism, occult meditation and various non-western medicines and theories of healing.

Unlike the claims made about lifestyle in epidemiological texts and scientific medical journals, accounts of lifestyle in alternative/holistic texts are often characterised by language expressing certainty and fact. This is similar to the risk factor health promotion literature or the self-help and fitness industry texts discussed above. However, in the alternative literature far wilder and more extreme statements are made. See, for example, this claim that lifestyle is the cause of multiple sclerosis:

No Mystery
In Australia, one in 2000 people is diagnosed with multiple sclerosis. The allopathic view is that this is a mysterious disease of unknown cause, with no known cure. . . . In fact, MS is a disease of civilisation, unknown in primitive societies. As acupuncturist and homoeopath John Craine points out: 'Rice eating countries show very little evidence of MS; it is much more evident where wheat is the principal grain in the diet. Evidence also shows that MS is a syndrome of malnutrition, derived from a low nutritional diet; not lack of quantity but lack of quality'. MS is mostly spread, he says, in those areas where dairy products are predominant. . . . The three main lifestyle factors responsible for degenerative diseases are the modern diet, stress and lack of exercise.

... From clinical and anecdotal evidence there is no doubt that lifestyle methods are the appropriate approach for MS and if persevered with, there are good grounds for optimism.

(French 1994: 102)

This example also demonstrates another important feature of alternative/ holistic conceptions of lifestyle and health, that is a focus on nutrition and digestion. In alternative/holistic accounts of lifestyle and health, a focus on the ingestion of 'healthy' foods appears not to be driven by any functional imperative but, instead, to involve the consumption of symbolic meaning, control and individual reflexivity. Thus, like the self-help, fitness and beauty industry and contemporary health promotion, alternative/holistic texts often conceive of health as a lifestyle choice articulated in terms of self-identity and consumption (e.g. Inglis and West 1983; Campion 1996).

Ironically, as with the new public health which also espouses holistic notions of health and a broadening of focus, the alternative practitioners' focus on diet often seems to contradict their own arguments about recognising the relationships between all aspects of living and health. By focusing on diet or other alternative practices, alternative/holistic texts frequently end up espousing a narrow lifestylist perspective that is far from being holistic.

Alternative and holistic theories about the relationships between food and disease are rarely considered salient in medical circles (Hamilton *et al.* 1995). This is largely because of their non-scientific basis. This is a reflection of the distinction commonly made between lay knowledges and medical (scientific) knowledges:

[N]utritional scientists are particularly prone to interpreting this kind of dietary choice [alternative health] as an instance of the persistence of magical and mystical orientations in a contemporary, rational, scientific era but in the guise of modern science. They tend to dismiss the ideas associated with these alternative dietary regimes as mere food faddism and, in fact, a new form of superstition.

(Hamilton *et al.* 1995: 498)

Despite the differences between alternative/holistic and orthodox medical perspectives, they should not be considered as opposites (Wolpe 1990; Montgomery 1991; Lowenberg and Davis 1994; May and Sirur 1998). In an article about the metaphorical systems underlying contemporary ideas about disease Montgomery (1991) argues that biomedicine and holistic health are in fact quite similar in their approach to disease. Modern medicine retains ideas about disease stemming from traditional healing and older medicines (Greek, Islamic). These ideas also underpin many holistic modalities (Montgomery 1991, 1993). Furthermore, biomedicine has always contained holistic ideas about the environment and personal circumstances, and holistic health and biomedicine utilise similar imagery to make sense of disease.

Similarities between orthodox medicine and alternative therapies can also be seen in the way that health and illness are understood in terms of functional meaning (Crawford 1980). This is demonstrated on popular medical infotainment shows on television and in the accompanying magazines (such as *Good Medicine* or *Healthy Wealthy and Wise*). These shows and accompanying books incorporate alternative therapies such as homoeopathy, acupuncture or herbalism with orthodox medical advice. This incorporation is easily achieved because the same language is used to refer to illness states and similar explanations are often given. For example, an Australian monthly magazine called *Women's Health* has a regular page titled 'Nature's way' written by a naturopath who 'offers a holistic approach to treating your medical woes and improving your overall wellbeing' (December 1999: 115). In response to questions written by readers of the magazine, the naturopath offers 'natural' suggestions that are presented in a similar way to medical prescriptions. For example, in response to a letter asking for strategies to avoid catching winter colds in an air-conditioned office building, the naturopath offers the following advice:

> I'd recommend taking 3000–4000 mg of vitamin C daily which will strengthen your cells against bacterial invasion, and a garlic tablet each day to help stimulate your immune system. If you're serious about staying well, you'll also need to reassess your diet. Steer clear of sugar and refined carbohydrates, as they feed viruses and bacteria.
>
> (December 1999: 115)

In another example of the occasional blurring between lay and medical thought that was apparent in lay texts, alternative/holistic texts often cited scientific journal articles or used medical terminology. This is despite the fact that alternative/holistic medicine is not based on science. For example, in a pamphlet about gut repair and liver detoxification printed by a company producing and selling a detoxification programme, the company's claims are expressed using scientific terms such as 'inflammatory or toxic reactions', 'bacterial imbalances' and 'metabolic dysfunction' (Metagenics 1999). When describing the minerals and chemicals which are provided as tablets and powders in their detoxification programme they use terms such as 'predigested hydrolysed lactalbumin', 'fructo-oligosaccharides and 'medium chain triglycerides'. This pamphlet also cites medical journals such as *The Lancet* and *Archives of Surgery*.

Just as alternative and holistic writings on lifestyle and health are influenced by biomedical language and ideas, alternative/holistic ideas may influence orthodox medical practice. For example, some orthodox practitioners practise acupuncture, homoeopathy, massage and meditation (Easthope *et al.* 1998, 2000a, 2000b; Eastwood 2000; Pirotta *et al.* 2000). May

and Sirur (1998) argue that medical doctors practise alternative treatments (in their case homoeopathy) for a number of reasons: an interest in
esoteric and marginal treatments; a desire to avoid unnecessary iatrogenic
disease; and because their own experiences of using alternative treatment
for their patients suggest that it is helpful. While May and Sirur did not find
that the doctors in their study were affected by patient/consumer demand
for alternative treatment, other authors have written about this. Bakx
(1991), for example, sees consumer demand as the driving force behind the
increased popularity of alternative treatments. Easthope (1993) and Kelner
and Wellman (2000) expand on this idea to suggest that orthodox practitioners who offer alternative forms of treatment are tapping into a patient
demand for customised care that caters for the individual.

Conclusion

Medical understandings of lifestyle vary between different medical fields.
They range from reductive conceptions of lifestyle as isolated behaviours or
practices which have been identified as risk factors for disease to broad
biopsychosocial conceptions of lifestyle as everyday life, family, work and
personal relationships. It is apparent that within the texts reviewed, medical
conceptions of lifestyle from epidemiology and the new public health are
used to explain disease and health in populations whereas risk factor health
promotion and some mainstream medical conceptions of lifestyle are used
to explain disease and health in individuals. Figure 4.1 illustrates the key
features of each of the different medical and lay conceptions of lifestyle
identified in texts in relation to each other.

Despite the range of conceptions identified in medical texts, a number of
generalised characteristics of medical understandings of lifestyle can be identified. First, when medical texts refer to lifestyle it is nearly always in the
context of a discussion about non-biological, social determinants or contexts of disease and health. Conceptions of lifestyle provide an explanatory
framework that is used in medicine to explain and account for the social.
However, medical conceptions of lifestyle reflect the individualised understandings of the social found in orthodox medical thought. They focus on
individuals within their immediate social environment and rarely account
for structural or cultural factors such as gender, socio-economic status,
class, race, sexuality or ethnicity. This is in contrast to the sociological
approach to explaining patterns of disease and health in terms of lifestyle
which was described in chapter 2 (e.g. Abel 1991; Bunton and Macdonald
1992; Cockerham 1995; Link and Phelan 1995).

This individualised understanding of lifestyle is demonstrated in texts
where patients are described as having a certain type of lifestyle or as having
lifestyle risks (it is never acknowledged in medical texts that doctors also
have lifestyles or that their opinions about healthy lifestyles are variable).
Because medical conceptions largely ignore differences in how a healthy

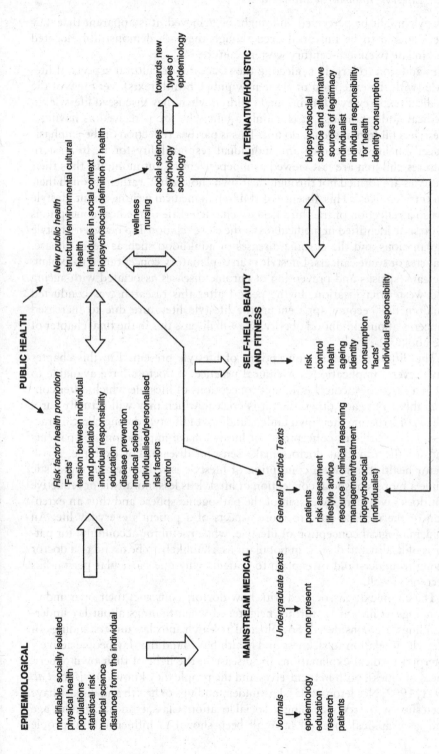

Figure 4.1 Overview of textual conceptions of lifestyle: visual summary illustrating inter-relationships between the different conceptions of lifestyle.

lifestyle might be perceived and might be achieved, it is apparent that they are assumed to be universal even though they are demonstrably located within late twentieth-century western culture.

In addition to largely neglecting the structural or cultural aspects of lifestyle (with the exception of some new public health texts), very few of the medical texts reviewed mentioned children when they discussed lifestyle. In medical understandings, it is mainly adults who are perceived as having a lifestyle; children, it seems, do not. This is partly a reflection of the emphasis placed on lifestyle choice and individual responsibility for it. In western cultures children are not viewed as independent or autonomous, thus their lifestyles are formed not through their own choices but, rather, through their parents' 'choices'. This absence of children in medical writing about lifestyle is also a reflection of the third general characteristic of medical conceptions of lifestyle identified in medical texts: the close relationship between lifestyle explanations and the chronic diseases of adulthood such as heart disease, diabetes or some cancers. Lifestyle is an explanatory concept used to explain the causes, risks and prevention of chronic diseases associated with ageing and western civilisation. In the period after this research was conducted children did become apparent in the lifestyle literature due to increased concerns about childhood obesity. We will discuss this in the final chapter of the book.

The different medical conceptions of lifestyle presented in this chapter have several implications for clinical practice. If doctors have available to them a range of medical (and lay) conceptions of lifestyle which differ considerably from each other, then it is unclear which they will actually enrol when constructing their own understandings of lifestyle during clinical practice. These different conceptions of lifestyle have implications for patients and for the way that doctors make sense of disease. For example, a risk factor health promotion conception of lifestyle is reductive and moralistic while a biopsychosocial conception of lifestyle is less moralistic or reductive but does involve an extension of the pathogenic sphere and thus an extension of the medical gaze to more aspects of a patient's everyday life. An epidemiological conception of lifestyle, while useful for accounting for patterns of health and disease in populations, is unlikely to be useful to a doctor trying to understand or explain to patients why one particular person has become unwell.

The complexity associated with how doctors construct their own understandings of lifestyle is further heightened when findings about lay understandings are considered. Sociological research into lay understandings of lifestyle in relation to sickness and health has found that lay people actively interpret medical explanations for disease in the light of their own experiences of illness, both in themselves and the people they know (Davison *et al.* 1991, 1992; Nettleton 1995). Lay understandings of health and disease have been shown to vary according to social location. Class, ethnicity, gender, age and geographical location have all been shown to influence how people make sense of sickness and health (Helman 1978, 1981a; Herzlich and Perriet 1987; Blaxter 1990; Green 1997). Lay people have also been shown to resist explanations for disease which do not sit well with their wider beliefs or which imply that they are responsible for their ill-health (Davison *et al.* 1991, 1992). Because of this, lay people will explain good health in terms of lifestyle but are more likely to explain illness in terms of factors outside an individual's control, such as fate, bad luck, susceptibility or biological causes such as a virus (Williams, R. 1983; Calnan 1987; Davison *et al.* 1991).

While doctors' understandings have not been studied in the same way as those of lay people, the limited studies which have been done suggest that doctors' understandings of lifestyle will also be influenced by their personal values, personal and clinical experiences and the views of patients (Atkinson 1981; Gaines and Hahn 1985; Arksey 1994). Thus when they make use of available medical and lay conceptions of lifestyle it will be in a complicated fashion. The next chapter addresses this issue through the presentation of interview and observation data. Using these data, we describe how individual medical doctors make use of various medical and lay conceptions of lifestyle when constructing their own understandings of the subject.

5 Doctors' understandings of lifestyle

Introduction

The previous chapter explored medical understandings of lifestyle through a thematic review of medical and lay texts in the form of typologies of lifestyle conceptions. This chapter continues exploring medical understandings of lifestyle by presenting the results of twenty in-depth interviews with doctors, observation of fifty-two doctor/patient consultations and eight participant observations of doctor/patient consultations.

The results presented in this chapter demonstrate that doctors draw on a range of different understandings of lifestyle when explaining different subjects including the risks and causes of disease, disease prevention, the social nature of ill-health, the social context of their patients, the management and treatment of illness, the maintenance of health and the delay of ageing. Understandings of lifestyle vary between different doctors, and individual doctors shift between different ways of talking about lifestyle as the issues they are talking about change. Furthermore, because doctors draw on non-medical conceptions of lifestyle their understandings of it blur the boundaries between lay and medical thought.

Lifestyle is also shown to be an explanatory concept that has limitations and benefits for doctors. It is limited by the individualised nature of medical conceptions of the social, the moralistic nature of many medical and lay conceptions of lifestyle and the fact that lifestyle models are unable to provide explanations for why some individuals develop disease. Lifestyle as an explanatory concept is of benefit to doctors because: lifestyle is an ambiguous concept which can be altered to account for a range of different situations; lifestyle provides doctors with a multicausal explanation for disease; lifestyle provides doctors with a framework to address the social (unlike other medical models of disease); lifestyle allows doctors to construct explanatory narratives which draw on everyday language to describe everyday practices; when talking about risk in terms of lifestyle doctors are able to present disease risk as containable and manageable.

A framework for the presentation of results: disease, illness and health

In their discourse doctors did not use a unified understanding of what lifestyle is, or how this might relate to disease, illness or health. Instead, they shifted between a range of different understandings of lifestyle as the topic they were discussing changed or as one particular way of talking about lifestyle ceased to be useful for them.

Although they often layered different understandings of lifestyle, it was nevertheless apparent that doctors spoke about it in six distinct ways that could be organised using the categories of disease, illness and health. Disease was used in reference to biological disorder and recognised disease entities; illness in reference to the social context of disease and the experience of being sick; health in reference to positive states of wellbeing and the maintenance of these states. The usual assumption underlying the disease/illness distinction (see Fabrega 1974, Dingwall 1976) is that doctors are concerned mainly with disease whereas illness is of concern to patients and lay people. However, we are arguing that when doctors talk about lifestyle they are concerned with all three: disease and illness and health. The different ways that doctors talked about lifestyle are summarised in Table 5.1.

After distinguishing between the different ways that doctors talked about lifestyle it was evident that many of their conceptions are familiar from the textual review presented in chapter 4. However, they also enrolled conceptions of lifestyle that were not evident in the textual review.

When doctors talked about lifestyle in relation to disease they enrolled those conceptions described previously as epidemiological and risk factor health promotion. When doctors talked about lifestyle in relation to illness, they enrolled biopsychosocial conceptions which were similar in some aspects to those conceptions of lifestyle identified in chapter 4 in the new public health, primary health care, general practice and the chronic illness literature. When doctors talked about lifestyle in relation to the maintenance of good health they enrolled conceptions of lifestyle found in risk factor

Table 5.1 How doctors spoke about lifestyle in different conversational contexts

---

When talking about disease:

1 Lifestyle as a determinant of disease

2 Lifestyle as a risk factor for disease

When talking about illness:

3 Lifestyle as a patient's social history

4 Lifestyle in relation to illness management and treatment

When talking about health:

5 Lifestyle as a commonsense prescription for good health

6 Lifestyle as a magic formula for good health

---

health promotion, the self-help, beauty and fitness industry and alternative medicine. They also drew on commonsense lay/folk conceptions of lifestyle that were not found in any of the lay or medical texts reviewed in chapter 4.

Lifestyle and disease

Lifestyle as a determinant/cause of disease

None of the doctors Emily spoke to claimed that lifestyle alone could cause disease. When they talked about lifestyle as a cause of disease their accounts were characterised by uncertainty and qualification. They talked about lifestyle in conjunction with causes/determinants emphasised in other medical frameworks such as biochemical models, germ theory, genetic explanations and psychological explanations.

When doctors described lifestyle as a cause of disease they were speaking about the diseases which in Australia (and the United Kingdom, Canada and the USA) have been the focus of highly publicised lifestyle-orientated health promotion campaigns, such as some cancers, cardiovascular disease, adult onset diabetes and to a lesser extent certain sexually transmitted infections (O'Connor and Parker 1995; Australian Institute of Health and Welfare 1998). When talking about lifestyle as a cause of these diseases, the conceptions of lifestyle which doctors used were similar to those in epidemiology and risk factor health promotion texts. For example, when asked to describe what they meant by lifestyle in this context doctors gave definitions that included reference to specific types of behaviours such as smoking, lack of exercise, unprotected sex, and injecting drugs. In the following dialogue, Dr G, a twenty-six-year-old female registrar, provides a clear example of this way of conceptualising lifestyle:

Emily: Are there lifestyle diseases?
Dr G: OK, yeah, well obviously there are a lot that you could mention but obvious ones would be heart disease, lung cancer and their relationship to smoking. That is probably the most obvious one. ... Um, diabetes, you know, cerebrovascular disease, peripheral vascular disease. Most of these tie in with smoking but there are also other unhealthy lifestyle things such as not getting enough exercise, high blood pressure. All those sorts of things add into most of them.
Emily: When you are thinking about those diseases are you saying that lifestyle is a cause of disease or that it's just an issue affecting how a person will experience the disease?
Dr G: Well obviously they are related to the person actually having the disease in the first place.

When Emily asked doctors why they associated these diseases with lifestyle, most stated that they had not learnt about this relationship from health promotion, which they described as being aimed more at patients than at doctors. Instead, they talked about epidemiological research and made statements such as 'These are widely accepted, the connections between lifestyle and these types of diseases' (Dr L). The registrar quoted above (Dr G) did suggest that the relationship between smoking and certain diseases seemed very direct to her because she had been working on a hospital ward full of respiratory cases nearly all of whom were middle-aged or elderly smokers. She attributed their respiratory disease to their cigarette smoking. Thus she implicitly acknowledged clinical experience as an additional source of her knowledge about lifestyle.

Despite using ideas about lifestyle and disease which were derived from (or at least very similar to) the reductive conception of lifestyle found in risk factor health promotion, the doctors (at least to a degree) overcame this reductionism by constructing complex aetiological narratives which describe lifestyle factors as only one element in a multifactorial aetiology. The construction of stories which explain disease, define the normal and the aberrant, and attribute causality and responsibility has until recently been associated with non-western cultures and lay people within western cultures (e.g. Foster and Anderson 1978; Kleinman 1980). However, medical anthropologists have demonstrated that biomedical knowledge and practice rely heavily on narrative (Good and Good 1980; Atkinson 1988, 1995). '[C]linical medicine as an institutional discourse both uses storytelling as a central facet of its professional procedures and produces stories by bringing certain kinds of social phenomena under the umbrella of medical expertise' (Epstein 1995: 20).

The construction of aetiological narratives that describe lifestyle as one of many causes of disease is an understanding of lifestyle informed by the web of causality approach utilised in epidemiology (Krieger 1994). However, this way of describing lifestyle as a cause of disease is also similar to examples described by authors writing about the process of lay epidemiology (e.g. Davison *et al.* 1991, 1992; Whittaker 1995). Lay epidemiology is the process whereby non-medical individuals use scientific information about lifestyle and disease in conjunction with their own observations of illness and disease and understandings of chance and luck to construct explanations for disease (Davison *et al.* 1992). Through this process they seek to render information about the causes of disease personally intelligible. While lay epidemiologists make use of medical information, the explanations and understandings of cause and risk they construct often vary from the statistical conceptions of risk and more closely resemble lay understandings of risk as danger (Kavanagh and Broom 1998).

In the following example Dr A, a female general practitioner in her mid-forties, while clearly describing lifestyle as a cause of disease, also establishes that it is only one factor among many which may result in the expression of disease:

Dr A: I think that lifestyle can be a cause of disease. . . . Now if we talk about coronary heart disease, the things that come together to cause that expression, to cause that disease, to cause something to develop, fatty plaques in your blood vessels, are their genetics, sedentary lifestyle, the fact they smoke, the fact they drink too much alcohol, maybe stress has something to do with it, and the fact that their diet has been, ah, full of animal fats and not enough complex carbohydrates. It's a combination of things that have caused disease to be expressed, many of which are lifestyle.

The most frequently mentioned additional determinant in many of the diseases doctors associated with lifestyle was genetics. They spoke about individuals having varying levels of susceptibility to the diseases associated with lifestyle because of 'their genetics'. This notion of an 'individual constitution' is far older than contemporary epidemiological ideas about lifestyle. It features in nineteenth-century medical texts and in twentieth-century understandings of immune systems and immunity (Martin 1994). It is also a feature of contemporary lay understandings of bodily imbalance (Peters *et al.* 1998).

Describing genetics as a difficult to assess but important contributing factor in disease aetiology is a useful strategy for doctors. Attributing disease to genetics suggests that diseases are actually predictable and that their development follows a set of rules; it is just that science has not yet decoded these rules.

As stated on p. 96, doctors frequently seemed to be uncomfortable about claiming that lifestyle actually causes disease. In their statements about cause and lifestyle they raised issues about uncertainty in medical knowledge about the causes of disease, and in this context the disease they mentioned most frequently was cancer. This is not surprising: despite intense medical efforts throughout the twentieth century, medical understanding and control of cancer remain minimal (Fox 2000). In the following example, Dr P, an oncologist in his mid-fifties, concludes that for most cancers there is no explanation:

Emily: How do you explain the cause of cancer to your patients? Do you talk about lifestyle as a cause?

Dr P: Well in the case of lung cancer, people with lung cancer know what caused it, nearly always. I had one lady just recently who had lung cancer at the age of seventy and when she came to see me she had a little cutting from a newspaper from 1968, which she had kept, which said 'Smoking does not cause lung cancer'. This had been her talisman all those years you see. So, a lot of people have blind spots and denial and that sort of thing. So, people won't accept it but in terms of what caused it a lot of people are very concerned to know whether there is a hereditary factor because they are

concerned about their children. And most cancers, as far as we
know, there isn't. Apart from a few cancers that definitely are, like
breast and in a few cases colon cancer and a few others. So, in those
cases you give them advice as to what should be done for their
children. That's the main reason people want to know. People often
ask and we have to say, 'We don't know'. I mean some cancers the
risk goes up with smoking but not as dramatically as for lung cancer.
The fact is that for most cancers we just don't know.

Discussions of uncertainty regarding whether the causes of disease could
be explained in terms of lifestyle were often focused on an individual case. It
was as though doctors could easily describe lifestyle as causing disease in the
abstract but when confronted with a 'real life situation' lifestyle arguments
were no longer as useful or perceived as desirable. There are two possible
explanations for this pattern. The first is that epidemiological arguments
about lifestyle factors and disease are arguments designed to explain patterns of disease in populations. They are not sufficient to account for most
individual cases. This is particularly apparent when a doctor has a patient
who develops a serious disease despite having a healthy lifestyle. In this
next example Dr C, a general practitioner in her early forties, was clearly
saddened and frustrated by her inability to explain the reason why one of
her patients had developed cancer:

Emily: Do you ever have patients come to see you who are confused about
        why they got seriously ill with a serious disease because they have
        been practising a healthy lifestyle?
Dr C: Well I can [think of one] actually. This happened to a woman that
        I know, who is actually around the same age as me. She recently
        came to see me about a sore in her mouth, an ulcer. And it turned
        out to be oral cancer. The prognosis is very poor and she probably
        has only a few months to live. She asked me why that happened
        and I had to say that we just don't know. She had never been a
        smoker or a drinker. She was very fit and healthy. Sometimes these
        things just happen and we don't know why.

Sontag (1978, 1989) has described the ways that an absence of medical
explanation for cancer contributes to the fear associated with the disease. It
was apparent in doctors' accounts, such as the one above, that uncertainty
about cancer is also stressful for doctors. This example is a particularly
interesting one because Dr C mentions that this patient was the same age as
her. She also mentioned in a later section of the interview that she had
known the female patient referred to above for some years. Emily noticed
during the interviews that when doctors could relate closely to a patient
who had developed a serious life-threatening disease, then they were less
likely to offer straightforward explanations and more likely to talk about

the unfairness and unpredictable nature of disease. This relates to a second possible explanation for doctors' reluctantce to describe lifestyle as a cause of disease in individual cases: a lifestyle explanation imputes personal responsibility for disease and doctors are reluctant to hold individuals responsible for developing disease, particularly serious life-threatening disease.

Lowenberg and Davis (1994) made a similar observation after studying a group of alternative health practitioners. These practitioners offered theoretical explanations for disease which imply that individuals are responsible for their own health. However, when talking about or to their own patients, these alternative practitioners were reluctant to hold them responsible for their own ill-health and offered explanations for disease which contradicted their earlier statements emphasising individual responsibility.

Dr O, an oncologist in her early forties, spoke about one of her patients, a man with recurring melanoma. In her account she differentiated between internal factors under an individual's control, that is lifestyle factors, and external factors that an individual cannot control. She went on to emphasise the unknown aspects of cancer aetiology and the strong influence of genetics, and this particular patient's view that his cancer was related to stress.

Dr O: I don't think it is always as straightforward as that. I think it is often multifactorial. Some people will smoke all their life but they don't get lung cancer. Some people get lung cancer who don't smoke. Some people get heart disease despite having a low fat diet, no family history, living a physically active sort of life and apparently having all these factors in their favour. But these things are intrinsic to them, other factors, external factors have an impact on it but there is still something within the genetic material that has a pretty strong influence as well. I've just got a fellow who's recently come to see me as a new referral because he has a relapsed malignant melanoma. He is very sure that his very stressful life in the last couple of years has contributed to that relapse and melanoma is something that we know has immunological sort of tie-ups. And probably things tie into both mental and physical stress and he has brought that aspect up very much of late. But just what the dominant factors are is difficult to tease out.

Another interesting feature of this account is the way that Dr O includes her patient's own explanation for his relapsed melanoma. While she does not seem to be giving his version of events much primacy, she is still taking it into consideration. In contrast to the way that many of the experienced general practitioners and the two oncologists interviewed seemed to take patients' explanations for their disease relatively seriously, the two youngest doctors who had only a few years' experience expressed doubt about the usefulness of listening to patients. In addition, when I reviewed medical textbooks about diagnosis I found that their authors frequently warned against paying much attention to patients' versions of events, describing them as inaccurate and self-serving (e.g. Nyman 1996; Talley and O'Connor 1996). Sociological research into this issue has found that doctors take patients' explanations more seriously if medical understandings and medical language are incorporated into them (Peters *et al.* 1998). Mention of patients' explanations for disease was common throughout the interviews, suggesting that anthropological research into doctors' understandings of disease which found that they incorporate their patients' version of events into their own explanatory models is relevant to these results (e.g. Good and Good 1980; Helman 1988).

When doctors talked about uncertainty and the causes of disease several phrased their discussion in terms of scientific discovery, suggesting that answers to questions about aetiology are 'out there' but just haven't been found yet. Some doctors suggested that further research would support current claims about lifestyle and disease. However, others suggested that further research might very well debunk current thinking about lifestyle and some diseases. Specialists were more likely than general practitioners to mention the need for ongoing scientific research into the relative importance of lifestyle in disease aetiology.

As cautionary tales to demonstrate the dangers of assuming lifestyle causes disease, several doctors talked about recent examples in medical thought where diseases which had been commonly assumed to be largely attributable to lifestyle factors had recently been identified as including bacteria in their aetiology. For example, Dr P, an oncologist with considerable experience as a research scientist and academic researcher, spoke about bacterial plaques in arteriosclerosis and helicobacter and stomach ulcers.

When Emily was talking to doctors she frequently asked them how they knew the things they claimed to know about lifestyle and disease. When asking these questions Emily was interested in how they would seek to legitimate their claims about lifestyle and whether they ever acknowledged any non-medical 'non-reputable' sources of knowledge.

The majority of doctors told her that they had read about lifestyle in relation to disease in scientific medical journals. The two youngest doctors looked at Emily strangely, surprised that this was even an issue. Dr F told Emily that 'Everyone knows about lifestyle and disease'. When she asked the doctors if they had learnt about lifestyle during their training many said that while they might have done so, they didn't really remember it. As more than ten of the twenty doctors Emily interviewed had been practising medicine for more than twenty years, this is not entirely surprising. Their medical training must feel like a long time ago. Importantly, it may also be a reflection of a medical school curriculum which does not focus on lifestyle. In the review of contemporary undergraduate medical texts (reported in the previous chapter) it was found that lifestyle issues received only minimal attention. As contemporary medical arguments about lifestyle and disease only grew to prominence in the mid- to late 1970s it is highly possible that they were not a feature of medical training at that time. Interestingly, while general practitioners also talked about making decisions about the relative importance of lifestyle in disease aetiology on the basis of published scientific research, they were far more likely than any of the specialists to say that they developed their own ideas about the importance of lifestyle in the cause of some diseases on the basis of their clinical experience. In the following example Dr R, a general practitioner in his early forties, describes his opinion about lifestyle and disease in terms of his own experiences with observing relationships between his patients' behaviours and their diseases:

Emily: Having talked about the multifactorial nature of many diseases do you still ever think of some diseases as being caused by lifestyle?

Dr R: Well I see a lot of patients who smoke and get a range of illnesses so I tend to think of those conditions as being caused by their smoking. I know that there are other issues involved like heredity and stress but I still see that smoking plays a large part.

Emily: What about heart disease, does lifestyle play a role there?

Dr R: Well again, it's difficult. There are people who eat chips and pies, have enormous beer tummies, drink beer and smoke like chimneys and then live to be eighty-three [laughs]. But in my experience many of my patients with heart troubles are smokers who carry a bit too much weight around the middle. They also tend to be stressed people.

In these accounts the similarities between doctors talking about their clinical expertise and lay epidemiology are especially apparent. In the example above Dr R. is constructing his own hypothesis about the causes of smoking-related diseases and heart disease based not solely on formalised medical knowledge but also on his own experiences and the experiences of people he sees in his practice. When considering general practitioners and epidemiological knowledge about the causes of disease these doctors are in a very similar position to educated lay people. If expertise is recognised as contingent and not as automatically granted with the title of doctor, it is likely that in certain situations and in relation to certain types of highly specialised epidemiological information many doctors are lay people. Current theories of lay epidemiology and popular epidemiology fail to recognise the liminal position of the general practitioner (e.g. Davison *et al.* 1991, 1992; Brown 1992). General practitioners are not scientific experts in the field of epidemiology and they are community members. As such they are not excluded from processes of lay epidemiology.

Another pattern, which frequently occurred when doctors were talking about uncertainty and the causes of disease, was that this topic, however phrased, was usually followed by a more up-beat and positive discussion where issues such as the value of medical research or the importance of lifestyle modification were emphasised. For example:

Emily: But do you ever have a patient who *has* been working really hard to take care of themselves for a long time but still gets really seriously ill? How do you make sense of that? Do they ever talk with you about 'why has this happened when I did everything right?'

Dr J (emphatically):   Yep. Yes, that happens quite frequently. There is no answer for that. All I can tell them is that I just don't know.

Emily: Is that difficult for you as a doctor to do?

Dr J: Yes it is. Because it makes you realise yourself how vulnerable you are. And that is what it really comes down to. We are all vulnerable. [She pauses.] But one of the things that I really enjoy about medicine is empowering people. The old style medicine was that we don't tell them anything. I don't like that approach and I never have done. To me it has always been 'what can I tell the person that they couldn't find out for themselves and that will help them to look after themselves?'

While Emily was only able to observe this strategy during the interview (it did not arise during observed consultations), she considers it would serve two functions for doctors in the context of a consultation. First, doctors like their patients to leave on a positive note feeling that something can be done about their current or potential condition. Patients like to feel this way as well (Guadagnoli and Ward 1998). Second, this strategy also serves to help the doctors feel in control and able to offer useful advice. When, in the example above, Dr J was talking about empowering people and helping them to look after themselves she spoke in a very positive and enthusiastic tone of voice, leaning forward and smiling at Emily. It was apparent that saying these things made her feel very good about herself and her role as a doctor. This was in stark contrast to the hesitant tone and worried facial expression Emily observed when she was talking about how difficult it is when she can't explain why a patient has become seriously ill and she is made aware of her own vulnerability. Medical uncertainty is emotionally and existentially challenging for doctors and patients. It raises questions about:

> [t]he meaning-fullness [*sic*] as well as the efficacy of physicians' efforts to safeguard their patients' well-being, relieve their suffering, heal their ills, restore their health and prolong their lives. . . . [I]t evokes the inescapably tragic dimension of medicine: the fact that all patients – and all physicians as well – are mortal.
>
> (Fox 2000: 409)

In the next example, Dr P moves almost immediately from saying that we don't really know what the causes of disease are to saying that we are not powerless in the face of disease because we can reduce risk (a much more reassuring statement).

Dr P: I often see patients who have cancer and they say, 'Well why have I got cancer? I do all the right things, I don't smoke and I don't drink a lot. I eat a good diet and exercise, and don't have a lot of stress, so why should I get cancer?' But I mean the thing is of course that we don't know the cause of lots of things. We know that these actions will reduce the risk, particularly of heart disease and to a lesser extent cancer, but nobody in the medical field pretends that if you adopt these things you'll never get any disease. Things happen which we don't know the cause of. On the other hand, it's very difficult in the public health perspective if you get up and say, don't do this and don't do this and do this and this and you'll reduce your risk of getting things by 3.5 per cent! Well most people would say, well why should I bother!

Interestingly, he also mentions that medical uncertainty about whether or not lifestyle factors are disease determinants needs to be kept from people, otherwise they would never make the lifestyle changes advised in health promotion and health education campaigns. This opinion that the uncertainty associated with risk factors should not be publicised is common within the health promotion literature. For example, Egger *et al.* (1993: 17) state that 'health messages in the media cannot afford to be accompanied by the types of qualifications usually found in academic scientific reports' because inconclusive data are vulnerable to selective interpretation by the target audience (e.g. smokers). Dr P was familiar with this perspective due to his long-term involvement in the development and implementation of health promotion programmes focused on lung, cervical and skin cancer. However, an assumption that patients are unable to cope with medical complexity was shared by many of the doctors interviewed. When speaking with Emily doctors frequently made statements which undermined the decision-making capacity of their patients. During the observed consultations the doctor often withheld information from patients, telling Emily later that most of them don't want to know all the 'maybes'.

Occasionally when doctors were talking about lifestyle as a cause of disease they used loose generalised notions of lifestyle as a type of gap filler. That is, they were using undefined ideas about lifestyle to explain disease aetiology in situations where there was no clearly established 'medical' explanation. For example, when talking about diseases such as asthma, some cancers or immune system disorders, doctors used the term lifestyle but rarely specified what this entailed. For example, Dr L stated: 'There are more diseases probably caused by lifestyle than we know about.' When asked to describe what they meant by lifestyle in such cases doctors often gave a very broad and diffuse definition which included factors such as the environment, pollution, stress and working conditions. These were quite different from the very focused and specific definitions that they gave when talking about lifestyle causing diseases targeted in health promotion campaigns such as heart disease or lung cancer.

The gap-filling approach was most popular among the few doctors who were comfortable to talk in a fairly relaxed, informal and generalised way about disease (older general practitioners and two oncologists). These doctors seemed less concerned about the 'why' of disease and more focused on the 'what to do' aspects (i.e. treatment and management). For example, during Emily's interview with Dr H he spoke about lifestyle in this particular way several times. In the following example he clearly describes lifestyle as a likely explanation for some situations where the determinants of particular diseases have not yet been identified:

Emily: You said earlier that lifestyle factors don't cause disease, that they are risks for disease. So does that mean that in your opinion lifestyle is not a cause of disease?

Dr H: Well it depends on what you mean by lifestyle a bit, doesn't it? I told you before that I think of lifestyle in a very broad way. In relation to saying does lifestyle cause disease, well there are huge gaps in medical knowledge still. I don't think that as doctors we adequately recognise the role of lifestyle in many diseases. Diet, environmental factors, pollutants. All the aspects of modern living really.

Lifestyle is a useful gap filler because it is an ambiguous concept and thus provides a very flexible explanatory framework. As a term, lifestyle has medical legitimacy owing to its use in epidemiology and public health. This allows doctors to talk about lifestyle and to be perceived as doing so in a scientific and medically informed manner, whether or not this is actually the case. This feature of lifestyle as an explanatory concept is clearly demonstrated in the following section describing how doctors talked about lifestyle as a risk factor for disease.

Lifestyle as a risk factor for disease

All of the doctors whom Emily interviewed spoke about lifestyle in terms of risk factors and prevention. Lifestyle as a risk factor for disease was usually mentioned very early in the interview when doctors were asked the question 'What is lifestyle?' It also arose when they were talking about the prevention of the diseases most frequently targeted in health promotion campaigns.

Doctors were far happier describing lifestyle as a risk for certain diseases than they were about describing it as a cause of disease. When asked why this was the case they said, 'In medicine we talk about lifestyle as a risk for disease, it isn't really a cause of disease' (Dr I); 'Risk is medical, it's from epidemiology, it's about the likelihood of something happening' (Dr U).

Epidemiological discourse provides concepts and terminology which are familiar to doctors and are widely accepted by them as representing a suitably medical approach to lifestyle. Doctors can claim legitimacy from epidemiology whichever conceptions of lifestyle they happen to be using at the time.

That doctors consider there is a distinction between risk and cause is clearly illustrated in the following example taken from Emily's interview with Dr K, a female general practitioner in her late forties:

Emily: You said that lifestyle can place people at risk of disease, what do you mean by that?

Dr K: Well, STDs for example. If you don't live a particular lifestyle, you don't get an STD, do you? Or diabetes, adult onset diabetes is the result of the unhealthy western lifestyle with a high fat, high sugar diet, alcohol and little or no exercise.

Emily: That's interesting. But before when I asked you if lifestyle could cause disease you thought that the causes of disease were multifactorial?

Dr K: Cause is not the same as risk. I mean we can't say that eating fatty foods will cause a heart attack because it's not that simple. But if a person has an unhealthy lifestyle with a bad diet and no exercise they will increase the risk of heart problems.

Despite often explicitly stating that they had derived their understandings of risk from epidemiology, the ways that doctors talked during the interviews suggested that in contrast to the usual epidemiological understandings, they understood risk in an individualised and personalised way to mean an individual's personal danger of disease. This is far closer to the ways that risk is represented in risk factor health promotion than it is to epidemiological conceptions (Petersen 1996; Kavanagh and Broom 1998). Furthermore, doctors' descriptions of risk were very similar to the generalised lay understandings of risk as danger that have been described by sociologists investigating lay perceptions of lifestyle and risk (Blaxter 1990, 1997; Douglas 1992; Popay *et al.* 1998).

When doctors were asked to describe why lifestyle risks such as smoking or exercise are the focus of so much medical attention while other risks for disease are rarely mentioned, they stated that lifestyle factors are social and thus modifiable whereas biological risk factors such as genetic predisposition or existing disease states are not modifiable. Because they view lifestyle factors as being modifiable risks that are the property of individuals (thus an individual responsibility), doctors frequently talked about lifestyle risk in terms of control. For example, they stated the importance of controlling risk factors for various diseases. They also said that educating and encouraging patients to control their own lifestyles is an important aspect of the role of a doctor. Williams and Boulton (1988) made a similar finding when they interviewed general practitioners about the role of disease prevention in general practice. Two examples of doctors talking about lifestyle in terms of risk and control are Dr G, a twenty-six-year-old female registrar, and Dr P, an oncologist:

Dr G: Obviously you know we try to do our best, like with diabetes. We try and get people to control their diabetes as well as possible so that their adverse outcomes down the track are hopefully lessened. You know, whether that actually happens or not is really hard to say but that's what we do. We try to promote people to have a healthy lifestyle, control their diabetes, have good blood pressure, control their weight, those sorts of things.

Dr P: There's a huge range of factors that affect people's risk of getting disease, to some extent. Are these able to change? I suppose that's where doctors would be interested. What factors and so on in life are changeable? You can't change their sex and you can't change their age even though those are risk factors. But you can change some of the others.

The doctors described lifestyle risks as being controllable risks. By this, they meant that explaining the risk of disease in terms of lifestyle offers them (and their patients) the potential to manage and control risks for disease. The perception that lifestyle risks can be managed and controlled was often described by the doctors as being in contrast to other types of health-related risk such as corporeal risk such as genetics (embodied risk) and environmental risk (e.g. exposure to pollutants) which do not offer doctors or patients the sense that they can be managed or controlled to the same extent. Kavanagh and Broom (1998) describe how women with abnormal cervical smear results (corporeal risk) strive to take control of their embodied risk through lifestyle changes such as reducing stress and eating a healthy diet. These women chose to interpret their risk in terms of lifestyle because it made them feel in control even though lifestyle risks have greater moral consequences than do embodied risks (Metcalfe 1993).

The way that doctors talk about controlling lifestyle risks also has a great deal in common with the narratives of control described in studies of people with a chronic illness. Williams (1984), Pierret (1993), Radley (1993) and Epstein (1995) all describe the importance of narratives of control for people affected by illness. When individuals become chronically ill they construct narratives which 'reconstruct the course of one's life so that it accommodates the illness by providing it with a genesis', and which make sense of life in the face of continuing or worsening disability (Radley 1993: 109). Stories such as these are important because they allow people to address the uncertainty associated with illness in the terms of 'their personal situation and their stock of common knowledge about health and illness' (Radley 1993: 109).

Doctors also strive to manage uncertainty about the causes and risks of disease by telling stories which emphasise that disease is predictable and controllable. Understanding disease in terms of lifestyle factors is an explanatory framework that easily allows for the construction of narratives of control. This way of interpreting the meaning that controlling lifestyle risks has for doctors is a very different one from the usual sociological perspective on this issue which is presented in terms of medical control of bodies and patients and as an indicator of increasing medical surveillance (Douglas 1990; Lupton 1993; Hughes 1994; Armstrong 1995).

Doctors' understandings of lifestyle risk are also personalised and individualised when they talk about acquiring information about a 'patient's risk factors' (Dr J) as a resource for clinical reasoning/diagnosis. This understanding of lifestyle risk is already familiar from the thematic review of medical texts in chapter 4. As described in that chapter, collecting information about a patient's lifestyle (though not necessarily 'lifestyle risk') was referred to in general practice textbooks as being a vital part of the diagnostic process (Thouless 1974; Hodgkin 1978; Gammon 1990).

During interviews several doctors spoke about using information about a patient's lifestyle risks to assist with diagnosis and the prediction of possible complications before surgery or treatment. General practitioners said that they would collect information from patients about their risk factors such as smoking, high blood pressure and exercise levels to help them make a diagnosis. The two youngest doctors interviewed, who were both working in a large public hospital, each mentioned that they collect risk factor information from patients before surgery. In all these cases lifestyle risks were seen as easily identifiable and as belonging to patients. For example:

Dr F: I think personally, at this stage, I just tend to think well 'this person has this condition'. You ask them about the risks and you identify a few of the risks and that's about as far as you go. You know what I mean?

This way of speaking about lifestyle and disease, as though lifestyle risks can be used as an indication of current or future disease, is the closest of all the doctors' accounts to the type of reductive understanding of lifestyle risk criticised by many sociologists and outlined in chapter 2 (e.g. Hughes 1994; Petersen 1996). Doctors are operating with a very individualised and personalised notion of the social when they talk about lifestyle in terms of risk factors. Three exceptions to this were two specialists who worked in oncology and one general practitioner with graduate-level training in epidemiology. These three doctors used a more socially embedded conception of lifestyle risk, speaking about employment and unemployment in addition to factors such as alcohol use and smoking.

When the doctors were talking about risk factors for disease and disease prevention they often spoke in a very prescriptive, advice-giving fashion. We suspect that the nature of the in-depth interviews was conducive to this type of advice giving because the doctors thought that Emily needed to learn about the connections between lifestyle and disease as she was obviously very ignorant (judging by her endless list of questions). Her observation of consultations, in contrast to the interviews, suggested that this type of advice giving is relatively unusual in this context. This is despite doctors' claims during the interviews that they do offer lifestyle advice during consultations.

The observation of consultations took place at a clinic in a very poor suburb where the majority of patients had a very low level of education; many were unemployed and many had substance abuse problems. When Emily asked the doctor (Dr I) why he rarely gave his patients any advice at all about modifying their lifestyle he told her that there are only limited opportunities during a doctor/patient consultation when patients are open to preventive lifestyle advice from their doctors and no such opportunity had arisen during the consultations. If given at other times, the lifestyle advice would either be wasted or make the patients defensive, thus ruining rapport.

Dr I's disinclination to offer lifestyle advice was also related to his strong awareness that most of his patients were not in a position to make substantial lifestyle changes. He worked at a practice in an area of socio-economic disadvantage and ran a methadone clinic. Furthermore, Dr I had different expectations regarding what constituted a healthy lifestyle for these patients. He told Emily that for many of his patients, 'they're doing a pretty good job when they stay off drugs, refrain from committing crimes and turn up on time for their medical appointments' (Dr I).

In contrast with Dr I, one of the GPs in a practice dealing mostly with university students claimed during interview that she frequently offered lifestyle advice to her patients. A former patient of hers, Emily had found that she offered her lifestyle advice during consultations. Her discussion of this issue during the interview revealed that, unlike Dr I, she had little awareness of the external constraints her patients might experience in terms of changing their dietary or exercise habits. For example:

Dr C: Well I think it's a lot to do with attitude really. For example when you look at diet. I will often tell people that it's cheaper to cook for yourself than to buy a take-away. And that's the type of thing that if you have the attitude and the information, that you can do it, you know. Lots more fruit and vegetables. Fresh food, low fat, low salt. Yeah.

A tendency for doctors to talk about disease in a reductive or exclusionary manner or to be ignorant about the social context of the behaviours and habits characterised as lifestyle factors for disease is a frequent topic in the sociological literature (e.g. Lupton 1993; Hughes 1994; Nettleton 1995; Petersen and Lupton 1996). Certainly when doctors are using ideas about lifestyle taken from epidemiology and risk factor health promotion they tend to use limited conceptions of what constitutes the social context of disease. These medical understandings about lifestyle operate with an emphasis on individual behavioural choices with little reference to structural, cultural or symbolic constraints on these choices. Furthermore, these conceptions of lifestyle are perceived as being universally applicable. There is no sense that what constitutes a healthy lifestyle might be quite different from one person to the next.

During interviews, when the doctors tried using conceptions of lifestyle from epidemiology or risk factor health promotion to explain why their patients persisted with unhealthy practices despite medical advice to the contrary, they were unable to find satisfactory answers in the discourses of epidemiology and risk factor health promotion. The only explanations readily available to account for unhealthy lifestyle choices these discourses are moralistic ones which explain these choices in terms of laziness, stupidity, ignorance or lack of self-discipline.

However, doctors only rarely explained lifestyle behaviours in these ways because they were unwilling to use negative or derogatory terms about their patients. This left them with little choice other than to declare that they could not understand some of their patients' lifestyle decisions. For example, Dr F became very frustrated when she talked about times when she could not understand people's lifestyle behaviours.

Dr F: I've been working on a ward that deals with respiratory illnesses, also in the outpatients' department. We say to people, 'You have to stop smoking or this emphysema, or bronchitis or whatever it is, will just keep coming back.' But they don't. They don't stop smoking. Instead they just keep showing up again and again and needing to be hospitalised. I just can't understand them. It's obvious that their smoking is making them really really sick but they keep on doing it.

The doctors involved in this research showed a general reluctance to talk about the impact of poverty and disadvantage on their patients' health. Doctors only occasionally raised the issue of socio-economic factors making it difficult for their patients to make suggested lifestyle changes. When asked a direct question about this issue all of the doctors acknowledged that socio-economic factors would impact on the lifestyle choices of their patients. However, they were very unsure about how this might work. Usually they ignored the part of a question that addressed lifestyle and told Emily in response that they always try to keep a patient's financial situation in mind when suggesting treatment or medication.

We suspect this reluctance stems from two factors. First, doctors have trouble connecting individual behavioural 'choices' with structural issues such as socio-economic status, race or gender, partly because they are not trained to do this during their medical degree and partly because they frequently subscribe to individualist ideologies which stress personal autonomy and choice (Pescosolido and Kronenfeld 1995; Belcher 1997; Neittaanmaki *et al.* 1999). Second, doctors who have no choice but to be aware of such issues because their practices are in poor suburbs or because they work with disadvantaged patients through the public hospital system feel that there is nothing they personally can do about this problem, so there is no point worrying about it.

This should not be interpreted as an argument on our part that doctors are not concerned with the social context within which their patients become unwell or experience illness. On the contrary, during this project we found that doctors are very interested and concerned with illness.

Lifestyle and illness

Lifestyle as a patient's social history

The capacity of lifestyle as an explanatory concept to provide a language and a legitimate medical perspective from which to talk about the social was valued by doctors. While other medical explanatory frameworks do include knowledge about the social (Kelly and Field 1994; Williams 2001), this is limited. Recognition of this is reflected in the traditional sociological assumption that doctors are only concerned with the biological (disease) and that the social (illness) is a matter of concern for those outside medicine (Atkinson 1995). However, in everyday clinical practice doctors are constantly faced with issues relating to the social causes and social contexts of ill-health, and lifestyle provides them with a framework to talk about the social.

In the previous section, we described the way that many doctors often offered a definition of lifestyle from risk factor health promotion when Emily asked them at the beginning of an interview to tell her what they meant by lifestyle. They certainly did so if they began the interview focusing on disease. However, many of the doctors answered this question by talking about taking a patient's social history: this is a long-established stage in a consultation where the patient is asked about family, work and how life is 'going along', and perhaps about the medical history of parents and other close relatives (Usherwood 1999: 17).

Social history taking provides doctors with a medically legitimate framework and a time in consultations when it is appropriate to talk about lifestyle in a biopsychosocial manner, as distinct from the often reductive conceptions of lifestyle found in health promotion and epidemiology. The notion that patients have a social history in addition to a medical history (a history of past medical care including previous diseases, medical procedures, medications, inoculations, screening tests and life events classified as medical such as childbirth or menopause) was an important aspect of doctors' understandings of lifestyle and of the social.

We have previously described how doctors use understandings of lifestyle as a resource in clinical reasoning by giving information about a patient's risk factors as a diagnostic device. However, when talking about lifestyle in terms of social history, doctors are using the concept to place their patients in a social context. This allows them to anticipate which medical measures might be appropriate but also heightens their awareness of illness, how their patient is experiencing sickness in the present or might experience it in the future. Johanson *et al.* (1998) made a similar finding in their study of life-style discussion in doctor/patient consultations. They found that lifestyle information such as professional life, family life, sleeping habits, housing, exercise, smoking, appetite and drug use is a valuable clinical resource for doctors. Such information indicates various measures which patients could take to improve their health, provides a social context for present health problems, and may indicate the need for medical treatment.

A key feature of this conceptualisation of lifestyle is an explicit distinction between the internal biochemical workings of disease and the external social and lifestyle factors that appear to impact on these internal processes. When doctors talked about lifestyle as social history they described it as an issue relating to illness rather than in terms of disease. At times several of the doctors interviewed expressed doubts about whether lifestyle was actually a medical issue because it seemed to refer to the social and the external rather than to the biochemical, the medical. For example, in the transcript excerpt below Dr O, a female oncologist, describes lifestyle as a non-medical issue:

Dr O: Lifestyle comes pre-medicine. I do go into a detailed history with each patient, which includes, um, obviously the medical reasons they have come along to see you but also their past medical history. And a fair bit about things like where they live and with whom, what their support structure is like, factors like alcohol and tobacco that have a fair impact in various cancers but also lots of other illnesses. And, um, their interests and pursuits, their work.

An important feature of this way of talking about lifestyle is that it requires asking questions rather than giving advice. In many of the other ways that doctors talked about lifestyle they were the holders of knowledge and they felt they imparted this knowledge to their patient. When talking about lifestyle as social history, doctors described gathering information about lifestyle from their patients.

Because taking a social history involved asking their patients questions but did not necessarily involve assessing the answers in terms of risk factors or of good or bad behaviours, talking about lifestyle in terms of social history is a time during a consultation when the doctor and the patient come closest to having a conversation, the difference being that the patient is unlikely to be given much of a chance to ask the doctor about his or her family, work or friendships (Johanson *et al.* 1998). In this way, asking social history questions can serve to build intimacy and rapport between doctor and patient (Savage and Armstrong 1990; Corney 1991; Usherwood 1999). This was demonstrated in the observed doctor/patient consultations: Dr I always began by asking his patients about their work and their family.

Rapport building is another positive issue associated with medical concern with lifestyle that sociologists rarely consider when they criticise doctors' interest in lifestyle issues as being a reflection of increased medical power and a means of increasing the number of aspects of everyday life considered to be of medical concern (e.g. Lupton 1993; Bunton and Burrows 1995; Petersen and Lupton 1996). Studies of patients' levels of satisfaction with a medical consultation show that there is a strong emotional component in a successful consultation (Beckman and Frankel 1984; Gabe *et al.* 1991; Buetow 1995). Many of the doctors interviewed or observed expressed the opinion that it was important to 'get to know your patients'. For example:

Dr A: Well I think about it [lifestyle] straightaway when a patient first comes to see me. I ask them about their habits, smoking, exercise and diet, I ask them about their family and their working life. If they're a student, because we see a lot of students here, I might ask them about exams or whether they are particularly busy at the moment. Um, I might ask if they are married or have a boyfriend, whether they have any children. That sort of thing. It gives you a chance to get to know them a bit.

Sociological theories of medicalisation are still very relevant when considering medical understandings of lifestyle in relation to illness. Doctors were drawing on biopsychosocial conceptions of lifestyle that stem from primary health care, some aspects of the new public health, general practice and the chronic illness literature (e.g. World Health Organization 1986; Charmaz 1987, 1990; Usherwood 1999). These are conceptions of lifestyle specifically designed to address social and emotional factors.

When doctors talked about lifestyle in a biopsychosocial way, their understandings of what lifestyle is and how it relates to illness were very broad. This feature of medical understandings of lifestyle is open to sociological interpretation in terms of increasing medicalisation because the wide scope of issues perceived to be lifestyle issues defines many areas of personal life as health related (Petersen and Lupton 1996: 5). Lowenberg and Davis have described how orthodox allopathic medicine operates with the doctrine of specific aetiology and thus a narrow pathogenic sphere. In contrast, holistic/alternative health, through an emphasis on the application of a health/illness paradigm to nearly every domain of life, represents an extension of the pathogenic sphere 'into lifespheres' previously outside this jurisdiction (1994: 585). Lowenberg and Davis (1994) argue from this observation that holistic/alternative medicine should be considered in some respects as an extension of medicalisation. When considering the way that doctors spoke about lifestyle when they were using biopsychosocial conceptions, it could be argued that these medical understandings of lifestyle also extend the pathogenic sphere and are thus medicalising.

The relationship between alternative/holistic medicine and a lifestyle framework is further demonstrated when doctors' accounts contained explicit references to holism, notions of wellness and an emphasis on the importance of looking at the 'whole person'. In the next example the oncologist being interviewed offers a wide-reaching definition of lifestyle:

Emily: What do you think about when you heard me saying the term lifestyle – what did you expect to be talking about?

Dr O: Lifestyle, um, socio-domestic factors, how you schedule your activities, both home and work, um your interests, your pleasures, your commitments. Things that might have changed over time in terms of your commitments and activities. Style of life but also pace of life. A very broad thing. . . . I do dislike the fact that doctors are thought to be non-holistic and I think that if you do the patient full service then you have to be interested in whether they've got heart disease or a child that's just left home in an unhappy state or whatever else and that if you're only interested in the tumour then you'll never get to grips with the patient and you'll never actually get them as well as they should be at any particular point.

Despite frequently speaking about the whole person, most doctors did not use conceptions of holism from alternative/holistic medicine. Dr D, a general practitioner in her mid-thirties with a growing interest in alternative treatments, and Dr S, a doctor who describes himself as a holistic practitioner, were the only doctors among the twenty interviewed who explicitly spoke about lifestyle using language and ideas from alternative medicine. Dr D talked about prescribing lifestyle practices such as yoga, a special diet or homoeopathy in the same way that orthodox practitioners might speak about physiotherapy or prescription drugs. Dr S on the other hand spoke at length about the ways that illness cannot be understood without taking a person's entire life into consideration. He used many examples that drew on his training in alternative medical practices such as herbalism, acupuncture, reiki and meditation.

Apart from Dr S and Dr D, when Emily suggested that a psychosocial understanding of illness in terms of lifestyle might have something in common with the alternative health approach the doctors denied this interpretation. Dr J became quite annoyed, as though she was being accused of quackery:

Emily: When you think about patients and their lifestyle and their health, do you find yourself having to place them in a broader social context to understand them? Do you have that information? Like their marital situation, their job, their family life, where they live?

Dr J: I don't, I ask. Quite often I don't know, I might never have seen the person before, so I ask . . . you have to look at the whole person.

Emily: What about alternative health, herbs, nutrition and things like that? . . . Do you talk about these issues with your patients?

Dr J: Um, only when they ask me about them. Because I have to say from my own experience that I have seen a lot of people dabbling in that area and quite a lot of them come back and say that it was very expensive and it didn't help. I am very sceptical . . . If it's straight diet then it's another matter. But dabbling in drops of this and drops of that is another matter. I haven't had a lot of experience at all of people being helped by that.

Which particular issues are considered to be issues of lifestyle that should be raised when taking a social history varied between different types of doctors. The obstetrician/gynaecologist, dermatologist and haematologist gave quite specific examples that could be clearly related to issues of disease (such as smoking, exercise and type of employment) while many of the general practitioners and the two oncologists included issues such as emotional state and relationship pressures. For example, they spoke about finding out if 'patients have someone around to look after them when they were too sick to do it themselves' (Dr H), and about care giving (making food, cleaning the house, helping with tasks such as bathing), social support and psychological factors such as stress, depression, having a reason to live and/or get better, family relationships and hobbies. For example, when Emily interviewed Dr I, after observing him in general practice consultations, she asked him about lifestyle questioning in the context of history taking. He emphasised that for him the major social issues were family situation, interpersonal relationships and work:

Emily: I noticed that you always ask your patients about their families?

Dr I: Yes. It works to build rapport because it shows them that I remember them and know what's happening in their lives but I do it for another reason as well. A lot of the time patients come to see the doctor because they are worried about things. It's called somatization. Psychological worries present as a physical problem. Family problems are an important aspect of that. [Reconstructed quotation from written notes taken during interview with Dr I.]

This example clearly demonstrates the issue mentioned earlier in this section: for doctors, talking to their patients about their lifestyle under the rubric of social history taking was important not just because of the bearing this type of information might have on their patients' state of health, but also as a 'getting to know each other' session.

Rural general practitioners or doctors who have long-term relationships with patients often socialise with them and are thus able to talk to them about their lives on the basis of first-hand knowledge. For example, Dr H, a general practitioner who worked for fifteen years in a rural area where he also had family living, told Emily that he considered his background knowledge about his patients and their knowledge about him to be both satisfying and useful because it encouraged better doctoring.

In contrast to this type of concern with building rapport through discussion of family, other relationships and external pressures, during a dermatology consultation Emily observed that Dr T restricted her history taking questions to behaviours associated with Emily's skin such as whether or not she had a habit of face touching or working with cooking oils. She did not ask any lifestyle questions about her work, relationships or stress. This line of questioning has far more in common with the second way that doctors talked about illness and lifestyle, which came up when they spoke about lifestyle in relation to illness management and treatment.

Lifestyle in relation to illness management or treatment

When doctors talked about lifestyle in terms of illness management or treatment, they did so in two different ways. The first was focused on the impact of a patient's lifestyle on the outcome and experience of treatment for an illness. An example of this understanding of lifestyle occurs when doctors speak about advising their patients to exercise after surgery, childbirth or enforced bed rest. This is not general lifestyle advice about the desirability of activity; it is advice based on expert knowledge about how to avoid blood clots and thrombosis.

In this way of talking about lifestyle, doctors draw on specialised knowledge about diseases and treatments and utilise a focused definition of lifestyle that refers to very particular behaviours or practices which are associated with particular treatments, symptoms or side-effects. For example, both the oncologists mentioned that patients undergoing radiotherapy and some forms of chemotherapy should be careful about going outside in the sun because they become photosensitive. General practitioners outlined the importance of not drinking alcohol when taking some medications such as antibiotics. Here lifestyle is related to managing situations in the present rather than the prevention of future ill-health. (However, there could also be a focus on a lifestyle change to alleviate a current illness and thus prevent it continuing in the future or even worsening, e.g. through diet and exercise in the case of diabetes.)

The second conceptualisation of lifestyle in terms of illness management or treatment concentrates on the impact of the treatment for disease on 'a patient's normal lifestyle'. By this doctors meant the way that patients would normally live their life. This conception of lifestyle is broad in scope but also tailored to the individual. Individuals are seen to have their own particular lifestyle that may include aspects such as employment, hobbies, household tasks, family responsibilities, personal relationships and driving a car. For example, patients with inflammatory arthritis will be asked how their pain is impacting on their ability to do the things they would normally do. The goal of managing the illness with medication is to try and get the patient back to a state where they can drive the car or go to the supermarket (their normal lifestyle). Unlike the first conception of lifestyle in terms of management and treatment, this way of talking about lifestyle is orientated towards the future and the present. In this version lifestyle does not impact on health and illness as much as health and illness impact upon lifestyle.

In terms of context, the first concept of lifestyle as management and treatment occurred very frequently in accounts from three of the specialists. Two oncologists (Dr O and Dr P) and a dermatologist (Dr T) were all used to dealing with patients who had long-term medical treatments. A common example of this was when doctors spoke about modifying diet to cope better with the effects of chemotherapy. Here, doctors are using specialist knowledge about the usual side-effects of chemotherapy and knowledge about interactions between the chemotherapy drugs and the body's ability to digest/excrete certain chemicals found in food:

Dr O: There are some factors that are going to help them get through whatever treatment is proposed. Whether it be potentially curative or controlling treatment, or just to reduce symptoms that are there at the time. .... Being sensible with alcohol when on chemo is important. Also there are some things that make people photosensitive. Particularly with radiotherapy and some drugs. Making sure people are aware and that they cover up when they go outside. Also, I always encourage them to try and maintain their interests and physical activities because when they're not able to get out and do things and be physically active because of a consequence of their illness or their treatment, if they've got a good level of fitness to start then they are not going to be so far down to have to pick up again.

Unlike the specialists who were familiar with managing chronic conditions or three older GPs who frequently worked with older patients and chronic illness, the two younger doctors, both of whom had only worked in a hospital setting, did not talk about lifestyle as a management issue. Several of the other general practitioners were also silent on the issue of lifestyle and illness management, preferring instead to emphasise that a wide range of effective drugs is available for the management of chronic conditions such as high blood pressure and asthma. An exception to this pattern emerged when Dr K, a general practitioner in her fifties, spent a great deal of time during interview talking about lifestyle changes being a far more effective management strategy than medication for some chronic conditions:

Dr K: Well most people know that they have to manage type two diabetes using diet and exercise so I suppose that's an example of lifestyle. And then there's asthma where we know it's important to keep fit by doing moderate exercise. Another good example is skin conditions. A lot of people don't realise that what they eat and what they bath with can have an impact on their skin. Skin conditions are one of the things that we sometimes can't do much for. . . . Yep, when you are talking about a chronic type condition then lifestyle issues like those can make a real difference. Those sorts of changes can help people to manage and will help that person as much as or in conjunction with treatment.

In the second way of conceptualising lifestyle in terms of illness management and treatment, doctors use their expert knowledge about the *outcome* of a particular treatment or surgery or disease to talk about the way this will impact on their patients' general experiences of day-to-day living. When doctors talked about this they frequently expressed concern about helping their patients to 'live as close to normal as possible'. This category included discussions of lifestyle where doctors spoke about limitations imposed by illness/disease/disability and patients' attempts to live a lifestyle which they considered to be 'normal for them' even if it might appear quite abnormal to other people (for example, using a wheel chair or a colostomy bag). Here the deployment of ideas and concepts from the chronic illness literature is apparent (e.g. Charmaz 1987, 1990; Radley 1993; Thorne 1993).

During the interview with Dr O she expressed concern about trying to achieve normality for her patients within the limits imposed by cancer and cancer treatments. The following example shows the overlapping nature of the different lifestyle accounts. It could also have been cited in the previous section to illustrate how doctors speak about lifestyle and social history:

Dr O: I do go into a very detailed history with each patient, which includes um, obviously the medical reason that they've come along to see you but also their past medical history and a fair bit about things like where they live and with whom, what their support structure is, factors like alcohol and tobacco that have a fair impact in various cancers but also lots of other illness, also their interests and pursuits, their work. What they are able to do at the moment, what they have been able to do previously and what they would like to continue to be able to do and even for the period of their treatment, whether it is likely that is going to be interrupted or not and whether they can have the expectation of getting back to a normal lifestyle for them.

Knowledge about the everyday lives of their patients is important for doctors when they are trying to help a patient rehabilitate after a serious accident resulting in bodily impairment. In this next example Dr H found his extensive background knowledge about a patient (Paul) whom he also knew socially to be invaluable when helping him put his life back together after becoming a quadriplegic in a car accident:

Dr H: I knew that what Paul wanted was to live on his farm, keep his farm running and stay in his house. So that's what we worked towards, him and I. He made changes to the farm operations so that he could run it with help, and they put in ramps and concrete paths to the sheds. And I worked very hard to help him stay well enough to do what he wanted to do. He had to get used to big changes in his lifestyle, really the whole family had their lifestyles changed.

When doctors talked about the everyday lifestyle of their patients they did so largely on the basis of their own clinical experiences of the ways that treatment or illness impact on the lives of their patients. Like the other ways that doctors talked about the social, this is an individualised understanding of it. While doctors told narratives about the way that certain individuals' lifestyle was affected by their illness, they did not talk in a generalised or abstract way about how gender, ethnicity, religion and social class affect the ways that people experience chronic illness or medical treatment.

Lifestyle and health

Lifestyle as a commonsense prescription for good health

In addition to using lifestyle as an idea to orientate discussion of the social aspects of sickness, doctors spent much time talking about lifestyle and health. For the doctors, health was a relative state which was influenced by ageing and which could be improved and maintained or which could deteriorate. Furthermore, when doctors talked about health they often described it as 'feeling well', indicating that their definitions of health include an emphasis on emotional wellbeing. This demonstrates that when doctors explain health in terms of lifestyle they use a far wider definition than a simple biomedical one where health is simply the absence of disease or infirmity. The terms used by doctors to talk about health were similar to those identified in studies of lay perceptions of health (Blaxter 1990).

Accounts which involved doctors telling Emily commonsense prescriptions for health which emphasised general lifestyle issues such as a 'healthy diet', 'keeping fit', 'managing stress' and 'achieving balance' between the different aspects of everyday life (for example, work, leisure, family life, intimate relationships, personal interests) were a feature in interviews and in the ethnographic work. The ideas about what constitutes a healthy lifestyle found in these commonsense understandings are strongly informed by popular ideas of achieving bodily balance in order to maintain general health and a strong immune system. In this example Dr C offers a commonsense explanation for health:

Dr C: Students often don't have the healthiest lifestyle. I think that a lot of the problems that patients come to see me about are lifestyle related. If people sleep and eat properly, get some exercise and refrain from pumping their bodies full of poisons then they tend to stay pretty healthy.

Such conceptions of lifestyle are not distinctively medical. While they are certainly informed by medical knowledge, so too are commonsense lay accounts of lifestyle and health (Blaxter 1990; Davison *et al.* 1991, 1992; Pierret 1993). This is a way of understanding health in terms of having a healthy lifestyle as opposed to understanding disease in terms of an unhealthy lifestyle. Doctors' stories about lifestyle and health represent a broadly commonsense view that living a healthy life is sensible because a person's state of health is related to the things they do in their life. They are not accounts about the cause of disease; nor do they usually argue that a healthy lifestyle will cure someone who already has a disease. Rather they are about staying healthy. For example, Dr L, a general practitioner, suggests that a healthy lifestyle can help a person to stay healthy but it won't cure disease:

Emily: Will a healthy lifestyle stop people from getting sick?
Dr L: Well it's impossible to say that really. I mean living healthily, with a good diet and keeping fit, minimising stress and such like will obviously mean that you are healthier and less likely to get sick. . . . For an already reasonably healthy person eating better and getting exercise will make them feel better. It's difficult to say it will stop them getting a disease though.

Most of the things that doctors said about lifestyle in a commonsense way might equally well have been found in the self-help literature in a popular magazine or suggested by someone's mother. Interestingly, whenever doctors were asked the source of this type of lifestyle knowledge they (as usual) cited evidence-based medicine or said they had read about it in a journal. Some GPs stated they had also acquired knowledge through clinical experience. Doctors never claimed to have acquired knowledge from health promotion. This is a reflection of their perception that health promotion is aimed at patients, not doctors. As doctors frequently utilised conceptions of lifestyle from risk factor health promotion when they were talking about lifestyle as a risk for disease it is apparent that they do acquire information from this source. However, when doctors were asked if they had ever learnt about health and lifestyle from sources other than medical sources (e.g. magazines, television or family members) their responses were mixed. Some said that they already knew about lifestyle so they didn't need to learn about it from anywhere else, while other doctors conceded that they might have. However, most seemed to think it was a very strange question to ask, implying that the source of doctors' knowledge was self-evident; it was medicine.

Commonsense accounts were often personalised, expressing an opinion that a healthy lifestyle is one that suits the individual as well as fulfilling the everyday criteria of a healthy lifestyle (e.g. a good diet and exercise). The following example is taken from the interview with Dr H. In this example he describes his own lifestyle, one which he considers to be healthy for *him*:

Emily: Do you have a healthy lifestyle?

Dr H: Well I try to. I don't work full days every day of the week any more so that I can spend time with my family as well as time for exercise and other interests. . . . Yeah, so I try to have a balanced lifestyle. Not just practice work all of the time. I went overseas last year and did a bit of research in the US. . . . And of course exercise is important. If you don't use muscles you just lose them and then everything can go. Karen [*wife*] and I both go to the gym and I walk the dog every day . . . keeping fit. And we all have spiritual side as well. I go to church regularly and I think that for me that is part of a healthy lifestyle.

This type of lifestyle account occurred frequently during Emily's own medical consultations. For example, during a consultation with Dr C where Emily complained about feeling tired all the time the doctor suggested that she make lifestyle changes:

Dr C: I think you should give it another week before we think about doing any tests. Probably you will be feeling much better by then. You could do some gentle exercise. Sometimes tiredness can be the result of inactivity. There are things you can do to boost your immune system and make yourself healthier all round. Eating green veg and fruit, and get plenty of sleep. Also you could try some vitamin C and echinachea. A good multivitamin never goes amiss.
    [Reconstructed quotation using notes taken after consultation.]

In general, commonsense prescriptions for wellbeing were characterised by moderation and were presented very much in terms of advice but not as certainties or as dictates. In contrast, the way that the doctors talked about a healthy lifestyle discussed below, as being a certain way to stay healthy in the future, was not characterised by either moderation or a recognition that such a lifestyle is not a guarantee of a long and healthy life. In addition, by arguing that a healthy lifestyle is a guaranteed way of achieving health and longevity, the doctors described below imply that it is a moral imperative.

A 'healthy' lifestyle as a 'magic' formula

Several doctors, all general practitioners, spoke about having a healthy life-style as though this were a *certain* way of controlling future health, a magic formula for future health. This way of explaining health in terms of lifestyle has elements in common with religious views on an ascetic lifestyle being a path to virtue and eternal life. These accounts were also quite evangelical because the doctors seemed to be trying to convince Emily that she should adopt a healthy lifestyle, make a kind of lifestyle conversion. This is similar to the way that proponents of alternative diets (organic foods, whole foods and vegetarianism) often speak about food and health. Hamilton *et al.* (1995) describe how the attitudes and beliefs of consumers of whole and health foods can be interpreted as having a magical or mystical orientation even when presented in the guise of rational science.

In addition, while doctors' advice about a healthy lifestyle leading to good health was positive and up-beat in tone it was also potentially moralising and censoring. Because they were expressed with such certainty and posited a healthy lifestyle as the cause of future good health, their implicit claims about individual responsibility for state of health were clear. This is apparent in the following example:

Dr E: Well a person's lifestyle is their health. The way that people live their lives is their health. . . . You see a healthy lifestyle, exercise and diet really are so important. By practising a healthy lifestyle people live longer and healthier.

Emily: So what type of relationship do you see between lifestyle and health? Is it a very direct one?

Dr E: Well it's direct in the sense that if a person lives a healthy lifestyle they are going to be healthy! If you mean in a causal sense it is more difficult.

Emily: You mentioned before that you have always exercised a lot. . . .

Dr E (interrupting):   Yes, yes I have always exercised, running, climbing swimming and cycling, marathons as well. People who don't exercise are really just asking for health problems later in life.

These accounts were usually offered by doctors who described themselves as having a strong personal belief in the importance of exercise and nutrition. However, in addition, as mentioned earlier, doctors also spoke about lifestyle in this way, in reaction to discussion of uncertainty about lifestyle and the prevention of disease, as though they felt that the interview needed to regain a sense of hope and action. The following example is taken from an interview with a GP in her late forties, also with a strong personal commitment to exercise:

Emily: So is it important having a healthy lifestyle?

Dr B: Well it's very, very important. I talk about it with every single patient who comes in here. Diet, exercise, smoking and drinking, safe sex.

Emily: Why is it so important?

Dr B: Well I guess it's a bit of a thing of mine. I really believe in it, especially exercise. I run everyday, ride my bike and swim. My kids all do a lot of exercise. It's vital really for staying healthy into the future. I can't stress it strongly enough really. ... I have always been active but now that we know so much about exercise and health I do it knowing that it really works.

When talking about control in this way of understanding lifestyle, the doctors described controlling their own health through lifestyle. In this personalised approach they often used words like believe or feel. This is in contrast to how they described controlling a patient's lifestyle. When they did speak about patients, several doctors described lifestyle advice as a valuable gift that they can give their patients to help them to control their own future or, in this next example, their own children's future. The doctors who talked about lifestyle and health in this way saw youthfulness and health occurring in conjunction with each other without the need to make any special lifestyle efforts. For older people to be healthy, however, many years of lifestyle vigilance were required:

Dr J: What you do with your health in your forties is what you will be in your sixties. That is my little saying because I really do believe that. If you just look the other way and drink a lot and smoke a lot, don't exercise ... then they are probably going to end up with diabetes at sixty-five, heart disease and not feel very well. Possibly well before that. So prevention takes place really from your age but most of us didn't know that in our twenties, whereas my children know that. They are on low fat diets now, in their twenties. So that is knowledge that they have that I didn't have. But I do know it now and I can take steps to do something about it, and therefore I feel that I can really stop the damage. And *that* is lifestyle thinking.

This example also demonstrates the way that these doctors perceived epidemiological research as 'proof' that a healthy lifestyle will result in future good health and longevity. This is a point of view familiar from the review of the self-help, beauty and fitness industry literature. Self-help books and articles about exercise and diet in women's magazines also see epidemiological data as 'proof' for arguments about the guaranteed positive effects of a healthy lifestyle (e.g. Hetzel and McMichael 1987).

As already mentioned, most of the doctors interviewed did not talk about lifestyle and alternative medicine or therapies. One doctor, however, identified himself as a holistic practitioner. His accounts of lifestyle were permeated with ideas and terminology from various alternative healing modalities and also enrolled scientific medical frameworks from various biomedical fields such as neurophysiology, psychology and immunology. His accounts of lifestyle and health emphasised controlling ageing through lifestyle. For example:

Dr S: What I'm really into now is anti-ageing medicine. . . . It's about total well-being, mind, body and spirit. Living in such a way as to prevent disease and achieve ongoing health and vitality by eating anti-oxidant foods, avoiding foods that cause ageing and toxification, taking nutritional supplements like drinks composed of marine algae, certain fruits. Learning and practising meditation, avoiding pharmaceutical and other drugs. . . . In anti-aeging medicine we take a preventive approach and see that ill-health is not inevitable. It's the result of the way we live.

Lifestyle understandings of health which identify the 'precursors of future illness' serve to 'deconstruct mortality . . . into a number of different diseases, each of which is "avoidable in principle" through the development of appropriate [i.e. medically or scientifically endorsed] "survival strategies" ' (Williams 1998: 441). Doctors who describe a healthy lifestyle as a magic formula for future good health are using a logic whereby 'death it seems only haunts those who are "careless of personal health" ' (Williams 1998: 441). This logic ignores (or neglects) the inescapable fact that everyone will eventually die of something.

The doctors interviewed were of course more aware of this fact than many lay people. They had been working with the evidence since they began their medical training. Nevertheless, for them, as for many non-medical people, the attraction of a lifestylist orientation was strong (Crawford 1984; Glassner 1989; Fitzgerald 1994). Unlike many lay people, however, doctors are unable to rely solely on this particular understanding of lifestyle because it is constantly contradicted by their clinical (and personal) experiences and because they also have access to other medical explanations for disease and health.

Discussion

Lifestyle provides doctors with a useful explanatory framework for a number of reasons. First, as demonstrated throughout this chapter, lifestyle is an ambiguous concept and thus provides doctors with a usefully flexible explanatory framework that can be altered to account for a range of different needs, including the need to explain the causes of disease, manage and treat illness and maintain good health.

Unlike many traditional medical explanatory frameworks (e.g. germ theory) that are clearly established and relatively stable, understandings of lifestyle have gained a place in the medical canon without ever being clarified or defined. Because of this ambiguity, lifestyle is a liminal medical concept where many discourses on the body, health, illness and disease meet and are contested. Thus the term lifestyle and ensuing perceptions about what lifestyle is and how this relates to disease, illness and health are open to interpretation within different medical disciplines and by individual doctors. Lifestyle also provides doctors with a satisfactory explanation for disease where aetiology is multifactorial and no straightforward explanations can be constructed using other medical models of disease. This was demonstrated when doctors used lifestyle as a gap filler in situations where there was no clear medical explanation for disease.

Second, understandings of lifestyle provide doctors with a widely accepted terminology and framework they can use to talk about the social context of disease and the social experiences of sickness (illness). Other medical frameworks do not provide doctors with a useful way of addressing the social. In the same way, lifestyle frameworks, because of their emphasis on disease prevention, are able to provide doctors with explanations not only for why people get sick but also for why they stay well. Again, this is in contrast to most other medical explanatory frameworks that are characterised by a focus on disease, not health.

Third, explaining health, disease and illness in terms of lifestyle also allows doctors to construct explanatory narratives which draw on everyday language and refer to everyday practices and behaviours. This has several advantages for doctors. Talking about everyday life helps to build rapport between doctors and their patients. Explaining disease, illness and health in familiar and accessible terms also serves as a useful heuristic device for doctors. In contrast to other medical explanatory frameworks that rely on esoteric language and concepts, doctors talk about lifestyle in accessible and familiar ways.

Finally, the way that doctors talk about lifestyle as a risk factor for disease provides patients and their doctors with a sense of control over the causes and risk of disease. This is in contrast to other types of disease risk that offer patients and doctors very little opportunity for management or control (for example, corporeal risk and environmental risk).

The interview, observation and participant observation data presented in this chapter also demonstrate that doctors understand the social determinants and contexts of ill-health and health in a far more individualistic manner than sociologists (e.g. Armstrong 1983; Calnan 1987; Blaxter 1990; Nettleton 1995). This is particularly apparent when they talk about lifestyle as a cause of or risk factor for disease. The individualistic way that doctors understand lifestyle is a reflection of the orthodox medical perspective which is based on assumptions of individualism and naturalism (Gordon 1988a).

While doctors did use broader biopsychosocial understandings of lifestyle to talk about illness and health these still focused on individuals within their immediate social environment (family, work, intimate relationships). None of the doctors explicitly addressed gender, ethnicity, race, social class or socio-economic status as factors which both constrain lifestyle choices and might result in differing perceptions of what constitutes a healthy or an unhealthy lifestyle; nor did they recognise that their own understandings of lifestyle are located culturally and historically. This suggests that doctors were assuming that the way they understood lifestyle was universally applicable. Kirmayer recognises this characteristic of medical biopsychosocial approaches:

> Without consistent attention to the experience of illness and the socio-moral dimensions of sickness, the 'biopsychosocial approach' of contemporary medical education will become just another technique for rationalizing the patient as a system of medical facts. Personality and stress will be variables duly noted and entered into the equation of the patient's distress, while disease remains the one solid fact about the person.
>
> (1988: 83–4)

As described in chapter 3, two negative implications of a universalistic and individualistic understanding of lifestyle are that such an understanding holds individuals morally responsible for their own sickness and is potentially discriminatory. Both of these problems were apparent in doctors' conversation about lifestyle. This was demonstrated most clearly when doctors talked about the causes of or risks for disease and when they talked about lifestyle as a magic formula for health.

Importantly, however, many of the doctors were reluctant to impute individual responsibility for disease. When talking about individual patients, they avoided using conceptions of lifestyle from moralising and discriminatory discourses such as those from the self-help, beauty and fitness industry or risk factor health promotion. Instead, they emphasised that they were uncertain about the nature of the relationship between disease and lifestyle. They preferred to say, 'We don't really know what causes many diseases.'

The results presented in this chapter also demonstrate that there are many similarities between doctors' understandings and lay perceptions of lifestyle in relation to health, illness and disease. When the doctors explained illness or disease in terms of lifestyle they integrated their own personal experiences of bodies, health and sickness with scientific medical information about lifestyle and disease. This is similar to the process of lay epidemiology (Davison *et al.* 1991, 1992; Brown 1992).

This blurring of boundaries between medical and lay ideas about lifestyle was also apparent when the doctors talked about lifestyle and health. For example, they often gave commonsense lifestyle prescriptions for health that varied according to their personal experiences and views on the relative importance of exercise and diet. This finding is similar to those of other sociological studies of doctors' perceptions of lifestyle in the context of disease prevention (Davies 1984; Boulton and Williams 1986; Williams and Boulton 1988).

It is also no surprise that doctors utilised lay conceptions of lifestyle and talked about it in a similar fashion to lay people. Anthropological and sociological research has demonstrated convincingly that doctors do not restrict themselves to medical ideas about disease and health. Instead, they make use of a range of medical and lay ideas (e.g. Helman 1988; Ben-Sira 1990; Shapiro 1990).

> [Research into medicine and medical knowledge has shown medicine to be] changing, pluralistic, problematic, powerful, provocative. What medicine proclaims itself to be – unified, scientific, biological and not social, non-judgemental – it is shown not to resemble very much. Those matters about which medicine keeps fairly silent, it turns out come closer to being central to its clinical practice – managing errors and learning to conduct a shared moral discourse about mistakes, handling issues of competence and competition among biomedical practitioners, practicing in value-laden contexts on problems for which social science is a more relevant knowledge base than biological science, integrating folk and scientific models of illness in clinical communication.
>
> (Gaines and Hahn 1985: 3)

Further, as discussed in chapter 2, many doctors are not experts in the fields of epidemiology and population health. Thus doctors cannot always be considered as medical experts and thus as distinct from all lay people. In relation to epidemiological research about lifestyle many doctors are in a similar position to well-educated lay people.

Lifestyle explanations for disease are far more open to non-scientific, folk and lay assumptions than are other medical understandings of disease. Lifestyle explanations have entered popular culture and have been highly publicised through health promotion and marketing campaigns. Furthermore, they use everyday language, refer to everyday practices and behaviours and contain a range of sociocultural assumptions about desirable behaviour (Hughes 1994). While other medical explanations for disease (e.g. genetic models or environmental models) are also imbued with sociocultural values, they are less obviously affected by such assumptions. Consequently, utilising lifestyle as an explanatory concept increases the opportunities for doctors to use folk, commonsense and other ideas and for lay and medical accounts about lifestyle to converge. Studies show that lay people use medical and scientific understandings of lifestyle in addition to folk understandings (e.g. Blaxter 1983, 1990, 1997; Calnan 1987; Pierret 1993).

The analysis presented in this chapter also demonstrates that individual doctors display considerable variation in the ways that they define lifestyle and explain sickness and health in terms of it. While each doctor's personal understandings of lifestyle were unique because of the influence of their personal values and experiences, several patterns of difference were apparent. Having expected to find differences between males and females, we were surprised when we could not discern any clear differences between them. Instead, the clear patterns of difference were between different types of doctors, namely among the specialists, between specialists and general practitioners, between the two young doctors and the other, middle-aged, doctors and, finally, between doctors of any persuasion who expressed a strong personal commitment to a healthy lifestyle and those who did not.

Among the specialists the clearest difference was between the oncologists (Dr O and Dr P), the gynaecologist/obstetrician (Dr M) and the haematologist on the one hand, and the dermatologist (Dr T) and the epidemiologist (Dr N) on the other. The first group of specialists displayed a range of different understandings of lifestyle and shied away from making moralistic comments or implying that individuals are responsible for the development of diseases associated with lifestyle. The second group of specialists relied heavily on the understandings of lifestyle from epidemiology and risk factor health promotion. They seemed largely unaware of the moral implications of these types of lifestyle understanding. In addition, neither of these specialists mentioned medical uncertainty about the relationship between lifestyle, disease and health. Instead, they spoke about medical knowledge about lifestyle as undisputed fact.

Apart from Dr T and Dr N, the medical specialists were more comfortable than other types of doctors (GPs and the two young hospital-based doctors) in talking about gaps in medical knowledge and in acknowledging medical uncertainty about the relationship between lifestyle, disease and health. In contrast, general practitioners were (as a group) less comfortable talking about medical uncertainty. This seemed to be related to the importance they placed on not painting a negative picture about the ability of medicine to 'make a difference' (Dr S).

This difference is interesting in the light of the second pattern of difference between general practitioners and specialists: the discussion of clinical experience. Specialists (and the two young hospital-based doctors) also made different claims for legitimacy than did GPs. When asked where they had acquired their medical knowledge about lifestyle, specialists all cited scientific research as their primary source. General practitioners also did this but in addition they claimed legitimacy for their medical knowledge on the grounds of clinical experience. Clinical experience was highly valued by general practitioners. Many of them began their interview by telling Emily for how many years they had been practising and where they had worked (geographical location, movement between practices, being a partner in their own practice). Specialists did not offer this type of information until they were asked about their background. Then they were more likely to tell Emily about their training than about their years of experience as a doctor.

Furthermore, many of the examples from their clinical experience which were cited by general practitioners suggested that the relationship between lifestyle and the development of disease was uncertain. Despite this, as discussed above, many of the general practitioners were uncomfortable when talking about medical uncertainty about lifestyle and were more up-beat than the specialists when stressing the importance of a healthy lifestyle.

The two youngest doctors (Dr F aged twenty-four and Dr G aged twenty-six) were very different from the older and more experienced general practitioners and specialists. Both of these doctors relied very heavily on risk factor health promotion understandings of lifestyle. Consequently, they were far more certain about the relationship between lifestyle and disease and far more censorious and moralistic when talking about their patients' lifestyles. Furthermore, neither of these doctors talked about clinical experience that cast doubt on risk factor health promotion arguments about lifestyle and disease. They had worked in a hospital only and for a very limited amount of time. Their attitude towards their patients was markedly different from the empathy and compassion frequently expressed by many of the general practitioners, two oncologists and one haematologist.

The final pattern of difference between doctors was between those who explicitly stated that they had a strong personal commitment to a healthy lifestyle (which they defined as taking exercise, not smoking cigarettes, eating a low-fat diet and reducing stress) and those who did not claim such a commitment. Those who told Emily that they were committed to a healthy lifestyle (GPs: Dr B, Dr E, Dr H, Dr J, Dr S; epidemiologist: Dr N) used understandings that emphasised a direct relationship between lifestyle and disease. Among this group were also the doctors who spoke about lifestyle as a magic formula for health.

Conclusion

The interview, observation and participant observation data presented in this chapter have shown that doctors do not use a unified medical understanding of lifestyle. Instead, doctors construct different understandings of lifestyle according to context. These different types of understanding draw on a range of different conceptions of what lifestyle is and how it relates to bodies, disease, illness and health. Many of these are familiar from the textual review presented in chapter 4. For example, doctors frequently cited the conceptions of lifestyle found in epidemiology and risk factor health promotion when they were talking about biological disease (e.g. Russell and Buisson 1988; Rose 1992; Rothman 1998). When talking about illness doctors used broad and wide-ranging understandings of lifestyle which drew on biopsychosocial conceptions similar to those identified in mainstream medical texts, in particular general practice texts, new public health texts and the chronic illness literature (e.g. Neighbour 1987; Scheingold 1988; Gammon 1990; Stewart 1995). When talking about positive states of well-being (health), doctors were unable to find suitable understandings of lifestyle within the mainstream medical literature or epidemiology. Instead they cited conceptions of lifestyle from risk factor health promotion and the lay discourses of the self-help, beauty and fitness industry (e.g. Rosenfeld 1986; Hetzel and McMichael 1987; Kowalski 1989). This is summarised visually in Table 5.2.

As can be seen in Table 5.2, doctors' understandings of lifestyle reflect the range of conceptions identified in the textual review. However, doctors also used conceptions of lifestyle that were not apparent in these texts (either medical or lay) when drawing on commonsense/folk conceptions or when discussing their personal practice of a healthy lifestyle. Medical knowledge in practice is not a direct reflection of formalised knowledge as found in texts (Wright and Treacher 1982b). In addition to scientific medical knowledge, the doctors who were interviewed and observed construct their understandings of lifestyle from their clinical expertise, their personal values and life experiences, and what they learn from their patients.

Many of the doctors' understandings of lifestyle reflect the individualistic and body-centred orientation of orthodox medical thought. They are often universalistic and rarely account for structural or cultural differences. Because doctors understand the social determinants of disease in terms of individual behaviour, they believe either explicitly or implicitly that people who become unwell with a lifestyle-related condition are individually

Table 5.2 The conceptions of lifestyle used by doctors when talking about lifestyle in relation to disease, illness or health

Different conceptions of lifestyle	When talking about disease	When talking about illness	When talking about health
Epidemiological	Yes		
Risk factor health promotion	Yes		Yes
New public health		Yes	
General practice, primary health care and chronic illness literature		Yes	
Self-help, beauty and fitness industry			Yes
Alternative medicine			Yes
Commonsense/folk			Yes
Doctors' own lifestyle	Yes		Yes

responsible for this situation. This was apparent when doctors talked about lifestyle as a cause of or a risk factor for disease. However, when talking about individual patients, doctors were reluctant to explain their sickness in this way. Instead, they actively avoided using ideas about lifestyle that implied that individuals are morally responsible for their disease.

Explaining disease, illness and health in terms of lifestyle has a number of advantages for doctors. First, lifestyle provides a useful explanatory framework for them because its meanings are ambiguous and thus flexible. Second, lifestyle provides doctors with a medically legitimate language and framework that they can use to talk about the social. Third, talking about lifestyle allows doctors to discuss everyday experiences and practices and to explain disease or health using everyday language. Fourth, understanding lifestyle as a risk for disease provides doctors with the sense that they can control and manage disease risk.

In addition, when doctors used conceptions of lifestyle that are not distinctly medical, their understandings blurred the boundaries between lay and medical thought. This also occurred when they claimed to be using an epidemiological (thus scientific/medical) conception of lifestyle risk but in fact were using conceptions more closely aligned with those from risk factor health promotion and processes of lay epidemiology.

In contrast to the image presented to the world by the medical profession of a unified, consistent and stable medical approach to disease (or the reflection of this image found in traditional medical sociology), doctors make sense of health, disease and illness in a complex, personalised, shifting and contingent fashion which draws on a range of different explanatory frameworks (Gaines and Hahn 1985; Helman 1985a, 1985b, 1988).

6   Reflections on lifestyle in medicine

Introduction

This book began by locating contemporary medical understandings of lifestyle within the context of medical explanatory frameworks in general. We argued that explaining health and disease in terms of lifestyle is not a new approach; however, the contemporary medical understandings of lifestyle which are the focus of this book differ from earlier medical (and lay) ideas about behaviours and health. They are a product of a particular place and time, and represent several key aspects of late twentieth-century thinking about the body and health, namely a concern with identifying and controlling risk, the increasing prominence of epidemiological multivariate analysis as a source of legitimate knowledge about the causes of disease, the self as project and a neo-liberal emphasis on personal responsibility for one's own health.

We also argued that in several western countries lifestyle-focused explanations for health and disease have become increasingly popular and widespread. This can be seen in medical fields such as general practice, public health, nursing and epidemiology (White 2002; Rothstein 2003), among policy makers and governments and across the popular lay media such as newspapers, magazines and television shows.

The apparent popularity of the lifestyle framework has been noted by many writers. As we researched the issue for this book we found commentaries on the lifestyle framework written by authors from a range of disciplinary backgrounds starting in the late 1970s with Crawford (1978, 1980) and increasing in number in place with the growing popularity of the lifestyle approach throughout the 1980s and 1990s (Skolbekken 1995; Hughes 1994; Pearce 1996; Førde 1998). S. Milner argues that by the mid-1990s with the expansion of epidemiological thinking about lifestyle and risk, 'instead of "lives" people now have "lifestyles" ' and 'private health has become public property' (1998: 318).

We conducted research to explore medical understandings of lifestyle in medical texts and the talk of doctors. As a rationale for our research we drew attention to several knowledge gaps. The first was the lack of research into the ways that individual doctors and doctors from different medical fields understand and apply concepts of lifestyle. The second was the lack of studies that empirically explore the interrelationship between lay and medical understandings of lifestyle. While lay understandings of lifestyle have been extensively studied, medical understandings have often been assumed to be self-evident and clearly separate from lay knowledges. Thus the inclusion of medical ideas into lay perceptions of lifestyle and disease has been investigated but the inclusion of lay ideas into medical understandings has largely been inferred.

This chapter presents our reflections on the results of the empirical research and a discussion about the implications of our research findings for sociological thinking about lifestyle as a medical explanatory concept and for medical knowledge and practice in general.

Reviewing the results from the empirical study

When we began this research we wanted to explore how lifestyle was being conceptualised in different medical fields, how individual doctors spoke about lifestyle and how lay and medical understandings of it might interrelate. Our results also allowed us to build a picture of the way that lifestyle was being used as an explanatory concept for health and disease in Australia (and other similar countries) during the 1990s.

When the medical texts reviewed in chapter 4 are considered it is apparent that, apart from a few isolated examples in the new public health literature, the majority display an individualistic understanding of lifestyle. For example, in epidemiological journal articles lifestyle was frequently conceived in terms of isolated behaviours or practices. Considered in this way, the cultural complexity and social variation of these practices and behaviours is absent and their context is erased. For epidemiological researchers, this way of understanding lifestyle is largely pragmatic. Research designs and the limitations in size associated with the publication of scientific research encourage epidemiologists to work within a narrow focus and to limit discussion in articles to the most relevant details (Link and Phelan 1995).

While epidemiology is reductionist in that it usually relies on creating categories of people or risk factors, epidemiologists are showing increased awareness of the ethical consequences of the epidemiological classification of risk and formulating more sophisticated modelling techniques which allow for greater complexity (Susser 1996; Syme 1996; Shy 1997; Plant and Rushworth 1998). This new epidemiological perspective views the individual as 'embedded in a seamless web of relationships, including cultural systems, social, economic, and political systems at the local, national and international levels' (Smith 1998: 57–8). There is also a slowly growing interdisciplinary awareness in the field of social epidemiology and disease prevention whereby sociologists, epidemiologists, geographers and biologists are coming together to investigate social inequalities in health (Blaxter 2000a). Examples are studies that: use epidemiological methods to challenge taken-for-granted assumptions about lifestyle risk factors (Ebrahim and Davey Smith 2000; Heslop *et al.* 2001); those that replace older conceptions of lifestyle or life chances with concepts such as 'social capital' or 'lifecourses' (Lomas 1998; Graham 2002); those that include lay views and those studies that explicitly address the previously gender-blind aspects of much lifestyle-focused epidemiology (Brimblecome *et al.* 2000; Denton *et al.* 2004).

Some public health texts (particularly those from the new public health) and mainstream medical texts such as those from general practice (sometimes drawing on the new public health) did use biopsychosocial understandings of lifestyle where individuals were described as being part of their immediate social environment (family, relationships, work) (Hasler and Schofield 1984; Jonas *et al.* 2000). However, the biopsychosocial model remains firmly fixed within a biomedical paradigm that emphasises individual care and the treatment of physical disease. It fails to adequately acknowledge the structural forces operating to affect the health of individuals and populations and the influence of culture on knowledge, actions and even perceptions about suitable behaviours (Knight 1997). New public health understandings of lifestyle, therefore, still suggest a far narrower and more individualised conception of the social than that advocated by many sociologists. Furthermore, studies of public health disease prevention programmes demonstrate that when these broader biopsychosocial understandings of lifestyle are operationalised the result is usually little different from risk factor understandings (Richmond 1997).

When individual doctors are considered, our research found they draw on a range of medical and lay ideas about lifestyle. Six distinct ways that doctors used lifestyle to talk about health, illness and disease were identified during analysis of the interviews. How doctors talk about lifestyle varies according to the issue they are explaining, and according to factors related to each individual doctor. These include the area of medicine in which a doctor works, level of medical experience and age. Whether or not doctors have a personal commitment to a healthy lifestyle also impacts on how they talk about lifestyle and how they perceive it as relating to health, illness and disease.

Some medical doctors displayed an individualistic and, to varying degrees, socially divorced understanding of lifestyle issues. This is clearly demonstrated in their discussions about lifestyle, the causes of disease, and lifestyle risks and in their evangelical accounts of a healthy lifestyle as a formula for good health. However, in many contexts doctors' understandings of the social seem to provide adequate explanations for disease or health within their usual setting, that is, the context of doctor/patient consultation. It is thus questionable whether a more sociological approach (i.e. a structural-cultural perspective) would be of benefit to doctors or their patients. An individualistic, socially isolated conception of lifestyle sits easily within the general medical perspective and within many wider cultural understandings about health and disease which also emphasise the biological nature of disease and do not locate health-related behaviours in a wider social or cultural context (Pierret 1993; Nettleton 1995). It appears likely on the basis of other research (e.g. Pierret 1993; Johanson *et al.* 1994, 1998; Blaxter 1997) that many patients would be quite content with this understanding of lifestyle as it is very similar to their own.

In some situations, however, such as when doctors try to understand why their patients do not make suggested lifestyle changes, their individualistic conception of the social context of health-related behaviours is an impediment because it cannot adequately account for the patients' behaviour. In these contexts doctors might find considerable utility in a more sociological perspective that locates lifestyle choices within a framework of life chances. For example, medical attempts to encourage disadvantaged groups to give up smoking repeatedly fail. Lawler *et al.* argue that this frequent failure is because for such groups smoking may 'represent a rational response to their life chances informed by a lay epidemiology' (2003: 266). Thus the most effective way to reduce smoking rates is to improve the general health and life chances of individuals. Whether or not individual doctors would be able to 'do anything' with this increased understanding about lifestyle and life chances is, however, debatable, given both the constraints of the doctor/ patient relationship and the possibly negative consequences of further medical influence on people's lives which would be occasioned by doctors asking their patients to locate themselves within wider structures of power and inequality.

In some contexts doctors did display a far more socially located understanding of lifestyle than would be expected, given some sociological writing (e.g. Petersen 1996; Petersen and Lupton 1996) and texts from the extreme end of reductive medical understandings of lifestyle (e.g. risk factor health promotion). These broader conceptions were apparent when doctors talked about lifestyle in terms of a patient's social history, for example describing employment, family, personal relationships, financial pressures, children, loneliness and life stage events such as 'empty nest syndrome' as being aspects of a patient's lifestyle. While from the perspective of 'surveillance medicine' (Armstrong 1995) this type of understanding can be considered an extension of the medical gaze and the sphere of medical concern and control, it could also be seen as positive evidence that doctors are transcending the biological reductionism of orthodox medical approaches to ill-health (Engel 1981; Hahn 1983; Germov 1997):

> The boundaries between health and disease, between well and sick are far from clear and never will be clear, for they are diffused by cultural, social and psychological considerations. . . . By evaluating all the factors contributing to both illness and patienthood, rather than giving primacy

to biological factors alone, a biopsychosocial model would make it possible to explain why some individuals experience as 'illness' conditions which others regard merely as 'problems of living'.

(Engel 1981: 598)

However, when using a biopsychosocial approach, doctors are still largely ignoring social structures, gender, ethnicity, inequality, cultural difference and historical and geographical location in their explanations. For example, none of the doctors mentioned or displayed awareness of cultural variations, ethnicity or even gender as compounding factors related to perceptions of what a healthy lifestyle is and constraints surrounding available lifestyle choices. Nor did they appear to recognise material constraints on lifestyles such as poverty and unemployment. When doctors talked about lifestyle they frequently did so in a universalising manner which erased the issue of difference by omission. The universalising nature of epidemiological research on lifestyle is recognised by sociologists (and some epidemiologists such as Marmot *et al.* 1978, 1991) and was commented on in chapter 2. However, a tendency to explain disease in terms of lifestyle in a universalising manner is not restricted to doctors. Lay people also tend to ignore cultural and gender differences when they talk about lifestyle and disease (Wiles 1998; Emslie *et al.* 2001).

In relation to medical texts, the results of our thematic review also demonstrate that a type of victim blaming is clearly apparent in texts from risk factor health promotion, some new public health texts and most general practice texts. For example, in several general practice texts patients were described as untrustworthy and as poor judges of what constitutes a healthy lifestyle (e.g. Gammon 1990). However, in relation to the doctors interviewed and observed for this project, the issue becomes ambiguous. These doctors were undoubtedly moralistic in many of the different ways that they talked about lifestyle. For example, when they talked about cigarette smoking, diet or exercise they frequently implied that a failure to change was the result of patients' laziness, lack of self-discipline, stupidity or inability to understand 'what's good for them'. In the case of doctors who spoke about health from an evangelical type of lifestyle perspective, the moralistic undertones were overt. They described health as being achievable through lifestyle practices such as exercise and diet, and thus implicitly placed all those who are not healthy in the position of having brought their sickness upon themselves. The two youngest doctors in particular and two female general practitioners with firmly stated personal commitments to a 'healthy lifestyle' frequently expressed their opinion that an unhealthy lifestyle was a type of personal failing. One of the younger doctors went to the extreme of claiming that smokers should be denied expensive surgical treatments for smoking-related illnesses if they continue to smoke. After she had reflected on this statement she changed her mind, saying 'it wouldn't really be fair to do that' (Dr F).

In many ways, however, the doctors demonstrated an awareness of the moralistic nature of many conceptions of lifestyle, and tried to overcome this problem. None of them used only one conception of lifestyle. While at times nearly all of them spoke about lifestyle in a moralistic or discriminatory fashion, these same doctors also expressed concern about any suggestion that people might be to blame for their lifestyle diseases. Most doctors denied that individuals' lifestyle can be the cause of their disease. They also seemed very reluctant to impute responsibility for their ill-health to their patients. Two oncologists, one haematologist and several of the general practitioners spoke of uncertainty as to the causes of disease and displayed great compassion and empathy towards their patients. These findings are supported by results from several other qualitative studies of doctors' views on disease prevention and lifestyle counselling (e.g. Boulton and Williams 1983, 1986; Williams and Boulton 1988; Johanson *et al.* 1994; Calnan and Williams 1995). For example, Williams and Boulton (1988) found that several of the doctors they interviewed about prevention in general practice considered that the lifestyle-focused approach to disease found in health promotion should be avoided by doctors because it was intrusive and moralistic. Calnan and Williams (1995) also found that many of the general practitioners they interviewed saw health promotion as a 'moral intrusion' and were sceptical about the efficacy of an understanding of disease which emphasises lifestyle (1995: 385–6).

In addition to victim blaming, other features often described in sociological writing about 'lifestylism' are the merging between conceptions of being good health and being beautiful, young and sexually attractive, the idea that good health can be bought and that a healthy body (read, young and sexually attractive) is a marketable one (Lupton 1994a). It was interesting to see that neither medical texts nor the talk of doctors reflect this aspect of lifestylism. In fact, the almost complete absence of any reference to 'looking good' or looking 'slim' or even looking 'healthy' was a marked feature in medical texts and doctors' accounts. The closest that doctors came to this perspective was when they spoke of a healthy lifestyle as a clear pathway to future good health.

However, the absence of a commodified understanding of lifestyle in medical texts and doctors' accounts is in itself significant. In both these discourses, it is apparent that medical understandings of lifestyle ignore the fact that practices associated with a healthy lifestyle involve consumption which, inevitably, 'is constrained by social and material contexts' (Nettleton 1995: 51). This feature of doctors' accounts was described in chapter 5 when we commented on the way that general practitioners took it for granted that their patients would be able to afford the costs associated with exercise and healthy foods, or to have the leisure time necessary for healthy pursuits such as exercise.

Our results also suggest that lifestyle is widely cited within some medical fields because it has a number of useful attributes for doctors and others attempting to explain health and illness. For example, it has the capacity to address the social and explain health as well as disease; it provides an opportunity to draw on commonsense ideas about health and illness; there is a perception among doctors that explaining poor health in terms of lifestyle allows people to 'take control' over their future health.

The term lifestyle derives considerable medical legitimacy from epidemiology and thus provides doctors with a medically acceptable framework to use when accounting for the social determinants of disease and the social context within which their patients experience disease (i.e. illness). This enabled doctors to use commonsense knowledge and present it to themselves (and others) as scientific medical knowledge. Sociological writers argue that medical understandings of lifestyle rely heavily on mathematical conceptions of risk and thus are merely an extension of the orthodox modernist scientific medical perspective. Certainly epidemiology, through its emphasis on scientific and rational methods of 'monitoring, measuring and regulating the population in the interests of improving health status' (Petersen and Lupton 1996: 27), is a flag bearer for science and modernity. However, one of the most significant findings in this research is that epidemiological conceptions of lifestyle and lifestyle risk have only varying levels of influence on other medical understandings of lifestyle. The differences in conceptions of lifestyle risk between epidemiology and public health (in particular risk factor health promotion) were discussed in chapters 1, 2 and 3 of this book. The wide range of understandings of lifestyle (other than epidemiological) which have imbued mainstream medical writings on the subject were described in chapters 1 and 5 (for example, understandings from the social sciences, nursing and welfare).

It was demonstrated throughout the interviews and observation that while claiming legitimacy from epidemiology and reputable scientific sources such as medical journals, in practice individual doctors' understandings of lifestyle also reflect a range of other influences. Doctors draw on non-medical conceptions of lifestyle, including commonsense and folk knowledges, personal experience, the self-help and fitness industry, paramedical ideas such as those found in the new public health (deriving from sources as varied as social welfare, nursing, sociology and psychology), subverted statistical understandings of risk (such as those used by lay people or in risk factor health promotion) and statistical understandings of risk from epidemiology. However, doctors only rarely used an epidemiological understanding of risk. Instead, they were far more likely to talk about risk as a personalised and individualised entity. That is, they spoke of probabilities and individual danger in addition to states of risk or no risk. This way of talking about risk is similar to conceptions identified in risk factor health promotion and in lay accounts (e.g. Blaxter 1997; Kavanagh and Broom 1998; Davison *et al.* 1991, 1992; Frankel *et al.* 1991; Pierret 1993; Blaxter 1997), but is not grounded in population health statistics. The interrelationship between medical and non-medical understandings in lay epidemiology is complex.

We argued in earlier chapters that many doctors are in a similar position to well-educated lay people when it comes to interpreting and utilising epidemiological understandings of lifestyle and risk. They can thus be considered lay epidemiologists themselves.

A lifestyle framework also allows doctors to explain why some people are healthy and others not, and how to maintain or improve states of health and wellbeing. A major attraction of a lifestyle approach for all those concerned about health is that it is an explanatory approach which also suggests a way of preventing disease (Le Fanu 1999: 313). Thus talking about lifestyle provides a setting for doctors to discuss the social determinants and social contexts of disease and issues associated with illness and with health. Whether or not it allowed them to do this successfully is debatable. However, as this is a feature lacking in many other medical models of disease such as germ theory it did seem to be useful for doctors.

Furthermore, because lifestyle risks are conceived of in terms of individual choice, explaining health, illness or disease in terms of lifestyle risk is seen by doctors to offer their patients the capacity to manage their risk of disease, as well as actively maintain or improve their health. Unlike other conceptions of disease risk which offer patients (and their doctors) little scope for personal control, lifestyle risks are seen by many doctors as a liberating concept, enabling patients to 'help themselves'. Here we see an example of doctors drawing on the empowerment rhetoric of the new public health.

As discussed in earlier chapters, Kavanagh and Broom (1998) make a similar claim about lifestyle risk from the point of view of patients. They found that women with abnormal cervical smear results often interpret this embodied disease risk in terms of lifestyle because this offers them strategies for the management and containment of risk (also see Lewis *et al.* 2003). The popular media, particularly women's magazines, also abound with examples of people who claim to have overcome poor health and disease through lifestyle changes. It is important to note, however, that in these examples lay people are often making magical claims about lifestyle as a sure-fire way of preventing future ill-health rather than more moderate statements about reducing risk. Thus the April 2006 edition of Australian *OK* magazine ran an interview with singer Melissa Etheridge who spoke about her treatment for breast cancer and her new 'healthy' lifestyle:

> I totally changed the way I eat. Also I think yoga is one of the best things a body can do and walking is amazing. I truly believe the changes I've made in my nutrition and lifestyle assure me I'll never see cancer again.

Our results suggest that at the time we collected our data, lifestyle was the preferred explanatory model among medical people for a limited group of diseases only. These were the diseases that have been the focus of health promotion campaigns following considerable epidemiological research into lifestyle factors, for example cardiovascular disease, adult onset diabetes and lung cancer. Even when talking about these conditions, the doctors in our study rarely used lifestyle as an isolated explanatory framework. Instead they used lifestyle explanations alongside a range of other medical explanations for disease such as germ theory and genetic explanations. Furthermore, when they were explaining health or disease in terms of lifestyle they did not restrict themselves to the conceptions of lifestyle found in epidemiology, risk factor health promotion, the new public health or self-help texts.

However, it does appear that a lifestyle risk factor approach is continuing to grow in popularity and is becoming more widely used in the fields of epidemiology, public health and disease prevention (including those parts of general practice and nursing focused on disease prevention). This type of lifestyle approach has entered 'commonsense, taken-for-granted' medical knowledge in these fields and appears to be widely accepted and supported. For example, Rothstein argues that the concepts of risk factor and healthy lifestyle as a way of preventing disease were the 'greatest revolution' in twentieth-century public health and preventive medicine. In the preface of his recent book *Public Health and the Risk Factor*, he states that 'the acceptance of risk factors has produced changes in public health and medicine as profound as those that resulted from bacteriology and the germ theory of disease' (Rothstein 2003: i). Lifestyle approaches to disease prevention have also entered best practice guidelines such as disease prevention guidelines for cardiovascular disease produced by governments, NGOs such the Heart Foundation and professional organisations such as the Colleges of General Practice in Australia, New Zealand and the United Kingdom. In Australia the Royal Australian College of General Practitioners endorse, a population health guide to behavioural risk factors titled *SNAP* (Smoking, Nutrition, Alcohol and Physical Activity) (RACGP 2004). *SNAP* provides GPs with information on risk factors 'that can be used to educate patients about the need to change their lifestyle' (RACGP 2004: 5).

The scope of diseases considered by medical practitioners to be caused by lifestyle factors may also be moving beyond cardiovascular disease, type two diabetes and lung cancer to include a range of other common cancers. For example, a study conducted by researchers from the Harvard School of Public Health and recently published in the *Lancet* argues that nine preventable risk factors are responsible for more than one-third of cancer deaths. The majority of these were lifestyle risks, the most damaging being smoking, alcohol use and low fruit and vegetable intake. Excess weight and lack of exercise were described as key risk factors for some cancers in wealthy countries such as the USA and unsafe sex resulting in transmission of the human papilloma virus was a leading risk factor for cervical cancer for women in low- to middle-income countries (Dania *et al.* 2005).

Despite the undeniable popularity of a lifestyle approach in some published medical texts, government policy documents and popular texts in the years after our data collection ceased we have observed a number of changes and possible challenges to lifestyle thinking that may lead to modification of its meaning or even its abandonment.

Changes and challenges to the lifestyle model

The constant discussion of genetics as a factor in the causes of disease throughout the interviews and in wider medical and lay thought provides evidence that genetic explanations for disease are becoming increasingly prominent (Davison *et al*: 1994; Willis 1997a; Henderson and Maguire 2000). Press reports and medical journal articles about genetic predisposition to chronic diseases such as heart disease suggest that lifestyle risks might increasingly be interpreted within a genetic framework (Davison *et al.* 1989; Richards 1993; Conrad 1999; Shostak 2003). The fields of epidemiology and public health are adapting lifestyle models of disease to include genetics. 'In academic research centres, government regulatory agencies, and some community-based organizations there appears to be a "growing consensus" . . . that gene-environment interaction plays a critical role in etiologies of human health and illness' (Shostak 2003: 2327–8).

Lifestyle arguments combined with genetic arguments are already used in explanations for some patterns of illness distribution such as the high rates of diabetes among Aboriginal Australians (White 2002). In some cases these explanations seem to merge the moralistic individual responsibility implications of lifestyle arguments with a type of genetic fatalism. For example, 'it is claimed that Aboriginal people have higher rates of diabetes because they freely choose bad Western foods such as potato chips, soft drinks and alcohol, for which they are genetically "not programmed" ' (White 2002: 4).

Instead of recommending lifestyle changes across the board doctors may come to advise individuals to adopt specific lifestyle regimens because they are seen to be genetically predisposed to developing various lifestyle diseases such as heart disease or adult onset diabetes (Richards 1993; Davison *et al.* 1994; Advisory Committee on Genetic Testing 1998). In a rather crude way this already occurs when doctors ask their patients about their family history in relation to such diseases. For example, family history is included as a conditional and predisposing risk factor in cardiovascular risk assessment tables such as Framingham scores. Cardiovascular risk assessment tables are based on studies that show that major risk factors such as high blood pressure, cigarette smoking, diabetes, low serum HDL cholesterol and advancing age are additive in predictive power (Wilson *et al.* 1998). Doctors ask patients about these risk factors and then use the tables to build several risk scores (i.e. relative risk, absolute risk, absolute short-term risk) for a patient. This score is then used to guide decisions about appropriate lifestyle counselling and the prescription of preventive medication (Grundy *et al.* 1999).

In Framingham scores conditional and predisposing risk factors such as a family history of premature cardiovascular disease are seen as potentially denoting a greater risk than that revealed from 'summation of the major risk factors' (Grundy *et al.* 1999: 1354). However, the 'quantitative contribution and independence of contribution to risk' of these factors are not clearly understood (Grundy *et al.* 1999: 1354). Other risk assessment tables such as the one used in the New Zealand best practice evidence-based guidelines place greater emphasis on family history and include people with genetic lipid disorders (such as familial hypercholesterolaemia or familial combined dyslipidaemia) in the group of people viewed as being at very high risk of cardiovascular disease (New Zealand Guidelines Group 2003).

Genetic explanations are likely to increase in popularity because they provide doctors with a very useful explanatory strategy. As they currently stand (i.e. not well understood) they serve as another useful 'umbrella' explanation to deal with uncertainty in a similar way to lifestyle models. They also sit easily with older understandings about the causes of disease such as 'bad blood' and race- and class-based understandings (Epstein 1995). Such explanations also continue the lifestylist emphasis on risk and are quantifiable and science based. As individualistic biochemical explanations, they sit well with the medical model and the general universalism and individualism of western medicine. The advent of gene therapy casts the continuance of current lifestyle explanations into further doubt. There would be no need for lifestyle changes if genetic predisposition could be 'corrected' (Anderson 1995; Williams 1997).

A second challenge to lifestyle models of disease prevention is the use of medication to lower biological risk factors such as blood sugar levels, blood pressure and lipid levels. Medication is also being promoted as a tool in weight loss and smoking cessation. Thus traditional lifestyle interventions such as low fat diets and exercise regimes now have to compete with pharmaceutical interventions. While medical professionals and lay people have expressed concern about preventive treatment using medication, these measures are strongly promoted by pharmaceutical companies and in many clinical guidelines for the management of smoking cessation, high blood pressure, adult onset diabetes and cardiovascular disease (Benson and Britten 2002; Lewis and Barton 2003; Lewis *et al.* 2003). Evidence from clinical trials also suggests that for higher-risk patients medication to lower blood pressure and lipid levels are more effective than lifestyle interventions in preventing disease (British Cardiac Society 1998; New Zealand Guidelines Group 2003). Several doctors in our study also stated that patients prefer drugs because they do not require changes in behaviours or habits.

A related and important issue that may or may not represent a challenge to lifestyle models is their limited applicability. In many instances the limits seem to be put in place by health professionals in practice. Throughout this research we have observed lifestyle being used to explain chronic diseases such as heart disease, states of good health and poor health and issues associated with chronic illness and some medical treatment. We did not observe lifestyle being used in discussion of children, psychological disturbances such as schizophrenia or acute disease states. Unexpectedly, we also found very little reference to sexually transmitted infections, hepatitis or HIV/AIDS. In relation to mental illness and children, we infer this absence to be closely related to the assumption that lifestyles involve choices and individual responsibility. Neither of these characteristics is associated with children or the mentally ill in western cultures. Furthermore, lifestyle arguments are still strongly associated with the prevention of heart disease (a disease of adults) and the types of behaviours or practices associated with adulthood, such as drinking alcohol or smoking cigarettes. However, in the time since the research was completed we have observed a considerable change in relation to children and lifestyle.

A rash of recent medical publications about childhood obesity and poor cardiovascular health in children and teenagers suggests that the lifestyle framework is being expanded to include children (Fulton *et al.* 2001; Golan and Weizman 2001; Malinas 2001). This concern has been reflected in the Australian popular press, Australian research funding and public health policy (Lupton 2004; NHMRC 2004). Australian children are being portrayed as fat, sedentary overeaters. Numerous stories in the print and television media have focused on the health risks for these children if they don't lose weight and the State and Federal Ministers of Health frequently make statements endorsing interventions aiming to increase physical activity by Australian children (Lupton 2004). Recently they released government plans for all Australian primary school children to be weighed once a year and for a daily hour of compulsory physical activity to be added to the school timetable. In 2004 the National Health and Medical Research Council released special funding for primary health care research that addressed a number of priority areas, one of which was childhood obesity. There are similar concerns about childhood obesity in the United States, China, Canada and the United Kingdom.

This expansion of the lifestyle framework to include children is interesting as adults (parents, teachers, doctors) are still being portrayed as the people who are ultimately responsible for children's unhealthy lifestyles. Parents in particular are urged to monitor children's behaviour and weight. They are also advised to facilitate 'healthy' food choices through shopping, packed school lunches and cooking and to increase the physical activity levels of the entire family in an effort to prevent further weight gain in their children and to form sustainable healthy habits (Edmunds *et al.* 2001). This continued focus on adults is also apparent in the way that health risks associated with overweight children are described. Being an overweight or obese child is described as concerning because it will impact on future health: some studies suggest that overweight children become overweight adults (Hoffmans *et al.* 1988; Must *et al.* 1992; Power 1997).

While this is the currently accepted medical position on this issue (Edmunds *et al.* 2001), other studies do not support this assumption (Abraham *et al.* 1971; Wright *et al.* 2001). Wright *et al.* used data from the

'Newcastle thousand families' study to explore the 'effects of childhood obesity and underweight on adult obesity and risk factors for disease' (2001: 1280). After excluding those subjects who met criteria for a metabolic syndrome associated with obesity and adjusting 'for adult percentage body fat rather than body mass index', they found that there is considerable evidence that 'fat adults were not fat children' (Wright *et al.* 2001: 1284). In addition they also found that the relationship between children's weight and adult disease risk is 'much less deterministic' than is often assumed.

> There was a high degree of variation between childhood and midlife in terms of fatness and no net increase in adult disease risk for overweight children or teenagers, despite children who were overweight at 13 being twice as likely to go on to be obese adults. This is probably because half of those overweight at 13 did not become obese adults while those thinnest in childhood who went on to be fat adults experienced the most adverse consequences.
>
> (Wright *et al.* 2001: 1284)

Thus this study suggests that being thin in childhood and then becoming obese as an adult is far more damaging to people's health than being an overweight child. The authors argue that interventions in childhood that aim to reduce children's body mass index 'may not benefit adult health'. Meanwhile underweight in childhood 'should still be the focus of concern since it offers no protection against adult obesity and is associated with increased risk of adult disease' (Wright *et al.* 2001: 1284).

In addition to studies investigating the relationship between weight in childhood and adult morbidity and mortality there is a recently renewed epidemiological interest in the relationship between the intrauterine environment, birth weight and adult morbidity (Hale *et al.* 1991; Lucas *et al.* 1999). The foetal origins hypothesis 'links low birth weight to chronic disease in adult life and proposes that adaptations by the foetus to promote survival under less-than-ideal conditions lead to persistent changes in structure and function' (Singh and Hoy 2003: 532). A number of studies show strong associations between small birth weight, weight gain in childhood and risk factors for disease in adulthood such as high blood pressure, central fat and lipid and glucose metabolism (e.g. Huxley *et al.* 2000; Ong *et al.* 2000; Sing and Hoy 2003). Such studies have a number of implications. In relation to social inequality they highlight the importance of nutrition for pregnant mothers and suggest that caring for mothers and young children may be an important intervention for improving adult health. It is well recognised that mothers in low socio-economic categories are much more likely to have low birth weight babies (Kelaher *et al.* 2003). However, the reasons for low birth weight and the mechanisms by which low birth weight is associated with adult risk factors is unclear. Studies in disadvantaged and malnourished populations suggest that low birth weight is associated with poor maternal health, young motherhood, maternal smoking and undernutrition. This implies that the problem could be remedied through strategies such as smoking cessation by pregnant women and improved nutrition. However, studies of well-nourished and otherwise healthy mothers suggest a strong association between genetic and postnatal environmental factors (Ong *et al.* 2000; Lawler *et al.* 2002). Thus some mothers who do not smoke and who have adequate nutrition also give birth to small babies and were often small babies themselves.

In relation to lifestyle arguments it is unclear whether or not lifestyle modification in children and adults such as low fat diets and exercise can compensate for low birth weight and overcome the tendency of low birth weight babies to gain weight and become obese in adulthood. Despite this uncertainty there are recommendations that low birth weight babies be recognised as being at higher risk of high blood pressure and adult obesity and be encouraged to pay close attention to their lifestyle as adults. For example,

> interventions to encourage a healthy lifestyle with well balanced diets and regular exercise to contain weight gain in adult life, must be given priority. People with low birth weight need to be especially targeted to maintain a modest adult BMI to reduce chronic disease risk.
>
> (Singh and Hoy 2003: 535)

The sociological critique of medical lifestyle understandings

The sociological critique of the lifestyle approach was outlined in the early chapters of this book. We argued that this critique stands as an important reminder to policy makers and governments that attempts to actually improve health outcomes will be constrained if they are limited to the narrow ideas about social determinants of health (i.e. lifestyle) found in fields such as epidemiology and health promotion. It points to the failure of lifestyle-focused health education programmes to produce lasting improvements in health and questions the assumptions about the nature of social causes of disease that underpin epidemiological research into lifestyle (Petersen and Lupton 1996; Ebrahim *et al.* 2000; White 2002). Thus the critique may also be viewed as a clash of ideological perspectives and a defence by sociologists of the role of sociology as a legitimate source of knowledge about health and disease.

Lifestyle approaches partially originated from sociology. However, the contemporary medical ideas about lifestyle found in health promotion, the new public health and texts from general practice and nursing draw on quite different ideological perspectives on health from most sociology's. Medical (in particular epidemiological, new public health and health promotion) understandings of lifestyle are underpinned by ideologies of individualism, autonomy, self-determination and rationality. The result is that health is no longer the state of not being ill but rather something to which one should strive, a moral imperative.

In contrast, sociological understandings of lifestyle in relation to health and broader social determinants of health are largely underpinned by ideas from materialist social theory such as Marxism and some feminisms that emphasise the relationship between social stratification, social structures, inequalities and physical health. The mainstream sociological perspective on lifestyle is that people's behaviours (lifestyle 'choices') are constructed and constrained within a broader framework of life chances. Instead of health being a matter of individual responsibility and self-discipline, it is more usefully viewed as a reflection of social organisation:

> There are a wide range of mediating social factors that intervene between the biology of disease, individual lifestyle, and the social experience shaping and producing disease. These range from standards of living and occupational conditions, to socio-psychological experiences at work and at home, of men and women's social roles, and of hierarchical status groups based on ethnicity. These factors, in turn, have to be seen against the background of the overall patterns of inequality that exist within specific societies.
>
> (White 2002: 2)

The sociological approach to lifestyle and health also has a moral component. However, this is not centred on individuals, rather it implies that governments have a responsibility for health because they have the capacity to reduce inequality and improve material conditions through housing and food standards and employment conditions (White 2002; Wilkinson 2005).

Medical explanatory frameworks which explain disease and health in terms of lifestyle are also described by sociological writers as being characterised by a range of features which have negative implications for those affected by diseases considered to be lifestyle diseases. Medical attempts to explain health and disease in terms of lifestyle have been described as reductive, socially divorced, moralistic, potentially discriminatory and a perpetuation of the medical tradition of explaining health and illness in a modernist science-based manner (Crawford 1980, 1984; Kaplan 1988; Richardson 1991; Bunton and Burrows 1995; O'Brian 1995). Furthermore, the medical approach to lifestyle (and wider cultural understandings of lifestyle, disease and health i.e. 'lifestylism' or 'healthism') has also been criticised for reflecting, supporting and perpetuating the commodification of bodies and health (Glassner 1989; Featherstone 1991; Williams 1998).

A key feature of the sociological critique of lifestyle is a defensive or even aggressively anti-medicine stance. Medicine and medical practitioners are described as controlling, dominant and implicitly dangerous or threatening (Fox 1993). They are also represented as having an incorrect understanding of the social determinants of health and illness (e.g. White

2002; Petersen and Lupton 1996). Consequently medical attempts to explain health and disease in terms of lifestyle are represented as incorrect, flawed, and fundamentally less worthy than sociological explanations (Blaxter 2000a).

> What we have here in effect . . . is a further challenge to medicine involving not simply a 'debunking' of medical 'truth' claims, but a more or less wholesale crediting to the sociocultural side of the balance sheet of the body and disease qua fabricated or discursive entities. . . . The net result is the 'advancement' of these particular sociological critiques, in the eyes of its exponents at least, vis-a-vis other 'rival' disciplines or bodies of knowledge such as medicine, and their claims to know and explain the world. A somewhat arrogant assumption or form of sociologism . . . based on an 'I know best ideology' in which sociologists' own particular version of *reality* is seen as somewhat superior to that . . . of the medical scientist.
>
> (Williams, S. 2001: 150)

Such a perspective tends to overemphasise the negative aspects of a lifestyle-focused medical explanatory framework for patients and other lay people while overlooking the potential benefits of medical ways of making sense of health and disease. As demonstrated in our research, while a lifestyle approach has many limitations it also offers a range of benefits for patients and for the doctors who use these ideas. 'In stressing the limitations of medical interventions the physical and social contributions of modern medicine are all too frequently ignored [by sociologists]' (Kelly and Field 1994: 36). Frank (1997) reminds the reader that while a lifestyle approach is not the solution to problems of chronic disease often touted by public health proponents, lives have been extended and deaths made easier through the application of disease prevention strategies emphasising lifestyle. Authors who write about the experience of living with serious and/or chronic illnesses stress the value of frameworks which can be used by medical and non-medical people to explain the cause of such conditions and which also provide people with the means for improving health and reducing uncertainty (Robinson 1993; Prior *et al.* 2000). On the basis of our research we suggest the critique should be expanded to include recognition of the complexity associated with medical knowledge and practice and the functional benefits offered to doctors by explaining disease and health in terms of lifestyle.

In relation to wider sociological characterisations of medicine, the results of our research provide further empirical support for the ongoing sociological debate about the usefulness of traditional sociological descriptors, such as the lay/medical distinction, the disease/illness distinction and the medical model (Strong 1979a, 1979b, 1984; Kleinman 1980; Lindenbaum and Lock 1993; Gaines and Hahn 1985; Atkinson 1995; Williams 2001). Traditional sociological characterisations of the medical approach to disease are bound together by the underlying assumption that medicine is a coherent, homogeneous and easily identified body of knowledge (Helman 1985a; Atkinson 1995). The results of our research have demonstrated that medical understandings of lifestyle are not homogeneous or coherent (see also Hansen 2003a). Our research also demonstrates that medical and lay ideas about bodies, health and disease are intermingled. The idea that such an entity as lifestyle exists and that a person's or a group of people's lifestyle can be used to explain their health is an idea which sits on the boundaries between medical and lay knowledge.

When doctors talk about lifestyle, boundaries are blurred between scientific and non-scientific understandings of lifestyle, between epidemiological, public health, mainstream medical, self-help, beauty and fitness industry, alternative medical and other popular and folk understandings. The lifestyle advice offered by doctors represents a shift in what constitutes medical advice and thus in the lines between expert and non-expert knowledge. The types of lifestyle advice offered by doctors in our study could all have been offered by pharmacists, nurses or lay people such as parents or teachers. Even the specialised understandings of lifestyle associated with the management of illness and treatment are not so 'medical' that they could not equally well be offered by nurses or paramedical workers such as physiotherapists.

Thus it is apparent that medical understandings of lifestyle, whether in medical texts or in interviews or observations of doctors, are clearly not neutral or even particularly scientific. To varying degrees this statement could be made about many aspects of medical knowledge and practice (Wright and Treacher 1982a, 1982b; Gordon 1988a). However, it is important to note that the doctors in our study draw the legitimacy for their statements about lifestyle from medical research, and even those claims made in the popular texts were often supported by references to scientific publications (see also French 1994; Campion 1996).

Davison *et al.* (1991, 1992) and Frankel *et al.* (1991) argue that lay attempts to make sense of disease and risk have a great deal in common with medical fields of symptomatology, nosology, aetiology and epidemiology. It can be seen in our fieldwork results that a similar claim could be made about the commonalities between doctors' and lay people's understandings of lifestyle. At times doctors are themselves lay epidemiologists. Other authors investigating doctors' explanatory models for disease have made similar findings about the heterogeneous nature of 'in practice' medical knowledge (e.g. Gaines and Hahn 1985; Arksey 1994).

This finding has interesting implications for the evidence-based practice movement. Evidence-based medicine (EBM) is a methodology for medical decision making which aims to help doctors to practise medicine in a more scientific manner by helping them to understand and critically evaluate medical literature and medical treatments on the basis of external clinical evidence from randomised clinical trials, systematic reviews and other available evidence. Despite some dissenting voices, EBM is now widely viewed as 'one of the central foundations underpinning the organization and provision of health care services' (Silagy and Haines 1998: ix). Doctors are encouraged to take the following five-step approach to evidence-based practice: (1) define the problem; (2) track down the information sources; (3) critically appraise information; (4) apply the information to your patients; (5) evaluate effectiveness (Sackett *et al.* 1997). Thus from a doctor's perspective EBM entails 'the conscientious, explicit and judicious use of current best evidence in making decisions about the care of individual patients' (Sackett *et al.* 1996: 169).

Gordon describes the development of evidence-based medicine as an attempt to make medical practice (art) more scientific (1988b). She draws a parallel between the increasing visibility of the patient through medical surveillance and the way that doctors are 'being asked to make their practice more visible' (Gordon 1988b: 257). The data presented in this book suggest that for many doctors, asking their patients about their lifestyle is a valuable clinical resource which they use for the purposes of diagnosis and disease prevention, management and treatment. As such, it involves the application of expertise. However, despite the emphasis placed on rationality and science by health promotion advocates (e.g. Pels *et al.* 1989; Grimshaw *et al.* 1995; Worral *et al.* 1997), the ways that doctors understand and apply conceptions of lifestyle seem far more closely aligned with the 'artfulness' described by Gordon (1988b) and Elstein (1976) than the 'science' represented as desirable by the Royal Australian College of General Practitioners (1998) or authors such as Sackett *et al.* (1997).

> The two types of clinical knowledge are linked to two dominant metaphors in medicine – 'art' and 'science'. Their relationship is often depicted as physicians learning 'basic science' principles (theory, universals), which they then 'apply' to the care of individual patients, which is where the 'art' comes in. . . . Metaphors and symbols notwithstanding, the literature on medicine documents that both medical science and practice are often neither very scientific nor very artful – even by their own standards.
>
> (Gordon 1988b: 260)

It is well recognised within medicine that many doctors find EBM and clinical guidelines difficult to apply in practice (Skolbekken 1998). Medical writers have generally assumed that this is because doctors do not know enough about the principles and strategies of EBM or because they have only limited access to clinical guidelines and research findings. Our research suggests that even when doctors access scientific evidence they may not interpret or apply it in a scientific manner. It was, however, difficult to tell in our study whether or not doctors would have used epidemiological information about risk and lifestyle in a manner more closely aligned with epidemiological intentions if it had been presented to them in a different way.

Both sets of results, the review of texts and interviews/observation of doctors, indicate that there is no unified medical understanding of lifestyle in relation to ill-health. In particular, the conceptions of lifestyle and the perceived relationships between these understandings of lifestyle and states of health and disease, which are found in epidemiology and public health, are only some of a range of approaches to lifestyle used by doctors. Furthermore, the distinctions between lay and medical understandings of lifestyle are blurred. As such, our research provides further evidence that the lay/medical distinction has limitations (Bury 1997; Kangas 2002). Furthermore, interview and observation data demonstrate that doctors do not restrict their attention to disease but are also very concerned with illness and health. This provides empirical support for the argument that the disease/illness distinction, while a useful sociological device (see chapter 1), can only suggest some of the ways that doctors actually work (e.g. Good and Good 1980; Atkinson 1995).

These issues – that doctors use a range of different models of disease; that they make use of lay knowledges; that medical practice is not a direct reflection of formalised written medical knowledge; that doctors include the social in their explanations for disease; and that they are very concerned with wellbeing and not just biological dysfunction – are all further empirical evidence that the medical model should be recognised as an ideal type and not as an accurate description of medical practice.

Conclusion

The conclusion reached is that our research provides support for many of the sociological claims about medical understandings of lifestyle that we outlined in chapters 2 and 3: for example, that these reflect and reproduce a range of sociocultural assumptions about health, bodies and desirable ways of living and that medical understandings of lifestyle reflect an individualised and personalised conception of the social which (unlike the sociological conceptions of the social) fails to recognise that lifestyle behaviours and practices are culturally embedded and materially constrained.

Medical understandings of lifestyle are in many ways universalistic and reflect the orthodox medical perspective which locates the causes of disease and health in the individual regardless of ethnicity, race, socio-economic status or gender. Furthermore, the sociological critique presents an accurate representation of medical constructions of lifestyle from the areas of risk factor health promotion, epidemiology and the new public health. The negative implications of these understandings of lifestyle for medicalisation and the emergence of new forms of disciplinary surveillance have been convincingly argued by authors such as Armstrong (1995), Bunton *et al.* (1995) and Petersen and Lupton (1996).

However, our research also suggests that sociological writing about lifestyle may need to be expanded to recognise complexity and variation within medical understandings of lifestyle, the dynamic nature of medical understandings of lifestyle and the benefits for doctors (and at times for their patients) offered by lifestyle as an explanatory device. The doctors interviewed for this research did not provide a unified version of the current 'medical facts' on lifestyle. Instead, interviews with individual doctors show that when asked to define lifestyle and to elaborate on its relationship with health and disease, they shift between a range of distinct (and at times contradictory) understandings of lifestyle according to conversational context, personal values, personal and clinical experiences and the views of their patients. As they do this, doctors are drawing on a range of different sources for their knowledge about lifestyle, including public health, knowledge and experience from their own medical sub-speciality, popular knowledges and personal experiences.

These results have wider implications for medical sociology because they challenge the widely used sociological distinction between professional and lay and the assumption underlying the majority of sociological investigations into lay knowledge, that medical knowledge is a stable and coherent point of comparison (see also Shaw 2002). While many areas of medical thought are quite different from lay understandings it is apparent in the data presented above that understandings of lifestyle and the related ideas about healthy or unhealthy practices blur the lay/medical divide. Using lifestyle as an explanatory concept increases the opportunities for doctors to use folk, commonsense and other ideas and for lay and medical accounts about lifestyle to converge.

We have also touched many times in this book on the differences between sociological approaches to explaining patterns of health and disease with reference to social factors and medical understandings of lifestyle. It is not clear how (if at all) these differences can be reconciled. Currently, sociology appears to play a very small role as a source of medically legitimate knowledge about the social determinants of disease. However, as demonstrated repeatedly over the previous chapters, medical understandings (derived from mainstream epidemiology, health promotion and public health) are limited in their capacity to guide disease prevention interventions and improve health because they focus on individuals and imply that self-discipline and knowledge are sufficient to change lifestyles and produce better health (Phelan *et al.* 2004). The danger in unpacking different explanations for health and disease and comparing them in terms of underlying ideological differences is that it can all too easily seem that one side is right and the other wrong.

We consider that sociology has a great deal to offer medical fields such as public health and epidemiology. Social epidemiology (discussed in chapter 2) and multidisciplinary approaches drawing on sociology and social epidemiology are likely to be the most productive way of trying to reconcile individual/biological understandings of disease with social/ materialist ones. 'Rather than trying to understand the social determinants of health from the very partial viewpoint of an individual discipline, it is necessary to follow the issues across interdisciplinary boundaries, wherever they lead' (Wilkinson 2000a: 581).

In order to understand patterns of health and disease more successfully we need research that recognises the limitations of the standard medical approach to illness and disease with its individualist emphasis, and of the standard sociological and epidemiological approaches where the individual is in danger of being seen as a mere confluence of structural forces or risks. To achieve this end, both medical and sociological researchers will need to work together and to understand the other's perspectives on the social determinants of health. As sociologists we need to abandon simplistic conceptions of medicine as a monolith focused on biology. Medicine is a complex set of knowledge and practices integrally influenced by ideas from other disciplinary fields and lay notions of health and disease. This feature of medicine is particularly evident in the medical models of lifestyle investigated in this book.

References

Abel, T. (1991) 'Measuring health lifestyles in comparative analysis: theoretical issues and empirical findings', *Social Science and Medicine*, 32(8): 899–908.

Abraham, S., Collins, G. and Nordsiek, M. (1971) 'Relationship of childhood weight status to morbidity in adults', *HSMHA Health Report*, 86: 273–84.

Abrums, M. (2000) ' "Jesus will fix it after a while": meanings and health', *Social Science and Medicine*, 50: 89–105.

Adelaide Conference (1988) *Report on the Adelaide Conference: Healthy Public Policy*. Second International Conference on Health Promotion, 5–9 April, Adelaide, South Australia: Joint Publication by South Australian Department of Community Services and Health and World Health Organization, Regional Office for Europe, Copenhagen.

Advisory Committee on Genetic Testing (1998) *Report on Genetic Testing for Late Onset Disorders*, London: Health Departments of the United Kingdom.

Alderson, M. (1983) *An Introduction to Epidemiology*, 2nd edn, London: Macmillan.

Altschuler, J. (1997) *Working with Chronic Illness*, Basingstoke: Macmillan.

Anderson, W.F. (1995) 'Gene therapy', *Scientific American*, 273(3): 96–8.

Angus, J., Evans, S., Lapum, J., Rukholm, E., St Onge, R., Nolon, R. and Michel, I. (2005) ' "Sneaky disease": the body and health knowledge for people at risk for coronary heart disease in Ontario, Canada', *Social Science and Medicine*, 60: 2117–28.

Annandale, E. (1998) *The Sociology of Health and Medicine: a Critical Introduction*, London: Polity Press.

Arcury, T.A., Quandt, S.A. and Bell, R.A. (2001) 'Staying healthy: the salience and meaning of health maintenance behaviours of rural older adults in North Carolina', *Social Science and Medicine*, 53(2001): 1541–56.

Arksey, H. (1994) 'Expert and lay participation in the construction of medical knowledge', *Sociology of Health and Illness*, 16(4): 448–68.

Armstrong, D. (1979) 'The emancipation of biographical medicine', *Social Science and Medicine*, 13(1): 1–8.

Armstrong, D. (1982) 'The doctor–patient relationship: 1930–1980', in P. Wright and A. Treacher (eds) *The Problem of Medical Knowledge: Examining the Social Construction of Medicine*, Edinburgh: Edinburgh University Press.

Armstrong, D. (1983) *The Political Anatomy of The Body: Medical Knowledge in the Twentieth Century*, Cambridge: Cambridge University Press.

Armstrong, D. (1988) 'Space and time in British general practice', in M. Lock and D. Gordon (eds) *Biomedicine Examined*, Dordrecht: Kluwer Academic Publishers.

Armstrong, D. (1993) 'From clinical gaze to a regime of total health', in A. Beattie, M. Gott, L. Jones and L. Sidell (eds) *Health and Wellbeing: a Reader*, London: Macmillan.

Armstrong, D. (1995) 'The rise of surveillance medicine', *Sociology of Health and Illness*, 17(3): 393–404.

Arney, W.R. and Bergen, B. (1984) *Medicine and the Management of Living: Taming the Great Beast*, London: University of Chicago Press.

Ashenden, R., Silagy, C. and Weller, D. (1998) 'A systematic review of promoting lifestyle change in general practice (GPEP project #324)', in *National Information Service: an Anthology of Literature Reviews by GPEP Researchers 1993–1997*, Adelaide, South Australia: Department of General Practice, Flinders University of South Australia.

Ashton, J. and Seymour, H. (1988) *The New Public Health: the Liverpool Experience*, Milton Keynes: Open University Press.

Atkinson, P. (1981) *The Clinical Experience: the Construction and Reconstruction of Medical Reality*, Aldershot: Gower.

Atkinson, P. (1988) 'Discourse, descriptions and diagnoses: reproducing normal medicine', in M. Lock and D. Gordon (eds) *Biomedicine Examined*, London: Kluwer Academic Publishers.

Atkinson, P. (1995) *Medical Talk and Medical Work*, London: Sage.

Australian Institute of Health and Welfare (1998) *Australia's Health 1998: the Sixth Biennial Health Report of the Australian Institute of Health and Welfare*, Canberra: AIHW.

Australian Institute of Health and Welfare (2002) *Australia's Health 1998: the Eighth Biennial Health Report of the Australian Institute of Health and Welfare*, Canberra: AIHW.

Backett, K.C. and Davison, C. (1995) 'Lifecourse and lifestyle: the social and cultural location of health behaviours', *Social Science and Medicine*, 40(5): 629–38.

Badura, B. and Kickbusch, I. (eds) (1991) *Health Promotion Research: Towards a New Social Epidemiology*, WHO Regional Publications European Series no. 37, Copenhagen: World Health Organization, Regional Office for Europe.

Bakx, K. (1991) 'The "eclipse" of folk medicine in western society', *Sociology of Health and Illness*, 13(1): 20–38.

Balint, M. (1964) *The Doctor, His Patient and the Illness*, 2nd edn, London: Pitman Medical.

Balint, M., Hunt, Joyce J.D., Marinker, M. and Woodcock, J. (1970) *Treatment or Diagnosis: a Study of Repeat Prescriptions in General Practice*, London: Tavistock Publications.

Bancroft, A., Wiltshire, S., Parry, O. and Amos, A. (2003) ' "It's like an addiction first thing . . . afterwards it's like a habit": daily smoking, behaviour among people living in areas of deprivation', *Social Science and Medicine*, 56(6): 1261–7.

Barsley, A.J. (1988) 'The paradox of health', *New England Journal of Medicine*, 318: 414–18.

Barsley, A.J. and Borus, J.F. (1995) 'Somatization and medicalisation in the era of managed care', *Journal of the American Medical Association*, 274(24): 1931–4.

Baska, T., Straka, S., Baskova, M. and Mad'ar, R. (2004) 'Effectiveness of school programs in tobacco control', *Central European Journal of Public Health*, 12(4): 184–6.

Bauman, Z. (1992) *Intimations of Postmodernity*, London: Routledge.

Beattie, A. (1991) 'Knowledge and control in health promotion: a test case for social policy and social theory', in J. Gabe, M. Calnan and M. Bury (eds) *The Sociology of Health Service*, London: Routledge.

Beaudoin, C., Lussier, M.T., Gagnon, R.J., Brouillet, M.I. and Lalande, R. (2001) 'Discussion of lifestyle related issues in family practice visits with general medical examination as the main reason for the encounter: an exploratory study of content and determinants', *Patient Education and Counselling*, 45(4): 275–84.

Beck, U. (1990) *Risk Society: Towards a New Modernity*, London: Sage.

Becker, M.H.A. (1993) 'A medical sociologist looks at health promotion', *Journal of Health and Social Behaviour*, 34(1): 10–23.

Beckman, H.B. and Frankel, R.M. (1984) 'The effects of physician behaviour on the collection of data', *Annals of Internal Medicine*, 101(5): 692–6.

Belcher, H. (1997) 'Power, politics and health care', in J. Germov (ed.) *Second Opinion: Sociology of Health and Illness*, Melbourne: Oxford University Press.

Ben-Sira, Z. (1990) 'Primary care practitioners' likelihood to engage in a biopsycho-social approach: an additional perspective on the doctor–patient relationship', *Social Science and Medicine*, 31(5): 565–76.

Benson, J. and Britten, N. (2002) 'Patients' decisions about whether or not to take anti-hypertensive drugs: qualitative study', *British Medical Journal*, 325: 873–7.

Bhopal, R.S. (1986) 'The interrelationship of folk, traditional and Western medicine within an Asian community in Britain', *Social Science and Medicine*, 22: 99–105.

Black, N., Rose, S., Davey, B., Gray, A., McConway, K., Popay, J. and Strong, P. (1984) *Caring for Health: History and Diversity*, Milton Keynes: The Open University Press.

Blackburn, C. (1992) *Improving Health and Welfare Work with Families in Poverty: a Handbook*, Buckingham: The Open University Press.

Blaxter, M. (1983) 'The causes of disease: women talking', *Social Science and Medicine*, 17(2): 59–69.

Blaxter, M. (1990) *Health and Lifestyles*, London: Routledge.

Blaxter, M. (1993) 'Why do victims blame themselves?', in A. Radley (ed.) *Worlds of Illness: Biographical and Cultural Perspectives on Health and Disease*, New York: Routledge.

Blaxter, M. (1997) 'Whose fault is it? People's own conceptions of the reasons for health inequalities', *Social Science and Medicine*, 44(6): 747–56.

Blaxter, M. (2000a) 'Medical sociology at the start of the new millennium', *Social Science and Medicine*, 51(8): 1139–42.

Blaxter, M. (2000b) 'Editorial note: Commentaries on Coburn. "The role of neo-liberalism" ', *Social Science and Medicine*, 52: 991.

Blaxter, M. and Paterson, E. (1982) *Mothers and Daughters: a Three Generational Study of Health Attitudes and Behaviours*, London: Heinemann Educational Books.

Bloor, M., Goldberg, D. and Emslie, J. (1991) 'Ethnostatistics and the AIDS epidemic', *British Journal of Sociology*, 24(1): 131–8.

Blumer, H. (1969) *Symbolic Interactionism, Perspectives and Methods*, NJ: Prentice Hall.

Bond, J. and Bond, S. (1986) *Sociology and Health Care*, Edinburgh: Churchill Livingstone.

Bordo, S. (1990) 'Reading the slender body', in M. Jacobus, E.F. Keller and S. Shuttleworth (eds) *Body Politics: Women and the Discourses of Science*, New York: Routledge.

Boulton, M. and Williams, A. (1983) 'Health education in the general practice consultation: doctor's advice on diet, alcohol and smoking', *Health Education Journal*, 42(2): 57–63.

Boulton, M. and Williams, A. (1986) 'Health education and prevention in general practice – the views of general practitioner trainers', *Health Education Journal*, 45(5): 79–83.

Bourdieu, P. (1984) *Distinction*, trans. R. Nice, Cambridge, Mass.: Harvard University Press.

Brandt, A.M. (1991) 'Emerging themes in the history of medicine', *The Millbank Quarterly*, 69(2): 199–214.

Bransen, E. (1992) 'Has menstruation been medicalized? Or will it never happen?', *Sociology of Health and Illness*, 14(10): 98–110.

Brimblecombe, N., Dorling, D. and Shaw, M. (2000) 'Migration and geographical inequalities in health in Britain', *Social Science and Medicine*, 50: 861–78.

British Cardiac Society, British Hyperlipidaemia Association (1998) 'Joint British recommendations on prevention of coronary heat disease in clinical practice', *Heart*, 80(supplement 2): S1–29.

Brooks, N.A. and Matson, R.R. (1987) 'Managing multiple sclerosis', *Research in the Sociology of Health Care*, 6: 73–106.

Broom, D. and Woodward, R.V. (1996) 'Medicalisation reconsidered: toward a collaborative approach to care', *Sociology of Health and Illness*, 18(3): 357–78.

Brown, P. (1992) 'Popular epidemiology and toxic waste contamination: lay and professional ways of knowing', *Journal of Health and Social Behaviour*, 33(3): 267–81.

Brown, P. and Mikkelsen, E. (1990) *No Safe Place: Toxic Waste, Leukemia and Community Action*, Berkeley: University of California Press.

Brubaker, R. (1984) *The Limits of Rationality: an Essay on the Social and Moral Thought of Max Weber*, London: Allen and Unwin.

Bruce, N. (1991) 'Epidemiology and the new public health: implications for training', *Social Science and Medicine*, 32(1): 103–6.

Buetow, S.A. (1995) 'What do general practitioners and their patients want from general practice and are they receiving it? A framework', *Social Science and Medicine*, 40(2): 213–21.

Bulmer, M. (1982) *The Uses of Social Research*, London: Allen and Unwin.

Bunton, R. and Burrows, R. (1995) 'Consumption and health in the "epidemiological" clinic of late modern medicine', in R. Bunton, S. Nettleton and R. Burrows (eds) *The Sociology of Health Promotion: Critical Analyses of Consumption, Lifestyle and Risk*, London: Routledge.

Bunton, R. and Macdonald, G. (eds) (1992) *Health Promotion: Disciplines and Diversity*, London: Routledge.

Bunton, R., Nettleton, S. and Burrows, R. (eds) (1995) *The Sociology of Health Promotion: Critical Analyses of Consumption, Lifestyle and Risk*, London: Routledge.

Bury, M. (1997) *Health and Illness in a Changing Society*, London: Routledge.

Byde, P. (1989) 'Contexts and communication for health promotion', in G.M. Lupton and J. Najman (eds) *Sociology of Health and Illness: Australian Readings*, 2nd edn, Melbourne: Macmillan.

Calfas, K, J., Long, B.T., Sallis, J.F., Wooten, W., Pratt, M. and Patrick, K.A. (1996) 'A controlled trial of physician counselling to promote the adoption of physical activity', *Preventive Medicine*, 25: 225–33.

Calnan, M. (1987) *Health and Illness: the Lay Perspective*, London: Tavistock.

Calnan, M. and Williams, S.J. (1992) 'Images of scientific medicine', *Sociology of Health and Illness*, 14(2): 233–54.

Calnan, M. and Williams, S.J. (1995) 'Challenges to professional autonomy in the United Kingdom? The perceptions of general practitioners', *International Journal of Health Services*, 25(2): 219–41.

Cambell, A. (1878) 'How to manage a baby: a lecture delivered in the City Mission Hall 6th June South Australian Public Library Adelaide', cited by K. White (1994) 'Nineteenth century medicine, science and values', in C. Waddell and A. Petersen (eds) *Just Health: Inequality in Illness, Care and Prevention*, Melbourne: Churchill Livingstone.

Campion, K. (1996) *Holistic Women's Herbal: How to Achieve Health and Wellbeing at Any Age*, London: Bloomsbury Press.

Cartwright, F.F. (1977) *A Social History of Medicine*, London: Longman Group.

Castel, R. (1991) 'From dangerousness to risk', in G. Burchell, C. Gordon and P. Miller (eds) *The Foucault Effect: Studies in Governmentality*, Brighton: Harvester Wheatsheaf.

Chambers-Clark, C.C. (1986) *Wellness Nursing: Concepts, Theory, Research and Practice*, New York: Springer Publishing Company.

Chang-Claude, J. and Frentzel-Beyme, R. (1993) 'Dietary and lifestyle determinants of mortality among German vegetarians', *International Journal of Epidemiology*, 22(2): 228–36.

Charles, N. and Walters, V. (1994) 'Women's health: women's voices', *Journal of Health and Social Care in the Community*, 2(6): 329–38.

Charles, N. and Walters, V. (1998) 'Age and gender in women's accounts of their health: interviews with women in South Wales', *Sociology of Health and Illness*, 20(3): 331–50.

Charmaz, K. (1987) 'Struggling for a self: identity levels of the chronically ill', *Research in the Sociology of Health Care*, 6: 283–321.

Charmaz, K. (1990) ' "Discovering" chronic illness: using grounded theory', *Sociology of Health and Illness*, 30(11): 1161–72.

Chavarria, F. (1989) 'Civilisation, diseases, time and space', in R. Krieps (ed.) *Environment and Health: a Holistic Approach*, Aldershot: Avebury.

Chessler, P. (1972) *Women and Madness*, New York: Avalon Books.

Chin, P. and Jacobs, M. (1983) *Theory and Nursing, a Systematic Approach*, St Louis, Mo.: C.V. Mosby Company.

Chopra, D.C. (1998) *Healing the Heart: a Spiritual Approach to Reversing Coronary Artery Disease*, New York: Random House.

Clough, P. (1992) *The End(s) of Ethnography*, Newbury Park, Calif.: Sage.

Coburn, D. (2000) 'Income inequality, social cohesion and the health status of populations: the role of neo-liberalism', *Social Science and Medicine*, 51(1): 139–50.

158 References

Coburn, D. (2004) 'Beyond the income inequality hypothesis: class, neo-liberalism, and health inequalities', *Social Science and Medicine*, 58(1): 41–56.

Cockerham, W. (2000) 'The sociology of health behaviour and health lifestyles', in C. Bird, P. Conrad and A. Fremont (eds) *Handbook of Medical Sociology*, 5th edn, Upper Saddle River, NJ: Prentice-Hall.

Cockerham, W.C. (1995) *Medical Sociology*, 6th edn, Englewood Cliffs, NJ: Prentice Hall.

Cockerham, W.C., Rütten, A. and Abel, T. (1997) 'Conceptualising contemporary health lifestyles: moving beyond Weber', *The Sociological Quarterly*, 38(2): 321–42.

Coffey, A. and Atkinson, P. (1996) *Making Sense of Qualitative Data: Complementary Research Strategies*, Thousand Oaks, Calif.: Sage.

Cohen, S., Halvorson, H. and Gosselind, C. (1994) 'Changing physician behaviour to improve disease prevention', *Preventive Medicine*, 23(3): 284–90.

Connelly, J. and Crown, J. (eds) (1994) *Homelessness and Health*, London: Royal College of Physicians.

Connor, S. and Connor, W. (1991) *The New American Diet System*, New York: Simon and Schuster.

Conrad, P. (1992) 'Medicalization and social control', *Annual Review of Sociology*, 18: 209–32.

Conrad, P. (1999) 'A mirage of genes', *Sociology of Health and Illness*, 21: 228–41.

Conrad, P. and Schneider, J.W. (1980) *Deviance and Medicalization: From Badness to Sickness*, St Louis, Mo.: C.V. Mosby Company.

Coreil, J., Levin, J.S. and Jaco, E.G. (1985) 'Life style – an emergent concept in the socio medical sciences', *Culture, Medicine and Psychiatry*, 9(4): 423–37.

Cormack, J., Marinker, M. and Morrell, D. (1992) *Practice: a Handbook of Primary Medical Care*, London: Kluwer.

Corney, R. (1991) *Developing Communication and Counselling Skills in Medicine*, London: Tavistock/Routledge.

Coulter, A. (1987) 'Lifestyles and social class: implications for primary care', *Journal of the Royal College of General Practitioners*, 305(305): 531–2.

Coward, R. (1989) *The Whole Truth: the Myth of Alternative Medicine*, London: Faber and Faber.

Crawford, R. (1978) 'You are dangerous to your health: the ideology and politics of victim blaming', *Social Policy*, 8(4): 10–20.

Crawford, R. (1980) 'Healthism and the medicalization of everyday life', *International Journal of Health Services*, 10(3): 365–88.

Crawford, R. (1984) 'A cultural account of health: control, release and the social body', in J.B. McKinlay (ed.) *Issues in the Political Economy of Health Care*, New York: Tavistock.

Crook, S., Pakulski, J. and Waters, M. (1992) *Postmodernization: Change in Advanced Society*, London: Sage.

Crossley, M.L. (2002) ' "Could you please pass one of those health leaflets along?": exploring health, morality and resistance through focus groups', *Social Science and Medicine*, 55: 1471–83.

Crossley, M.L. (2004) 'Making sense of "barebacking": gay men's narratives, unsafe sex and the "resistance habitus" ', *British Journal of Social Psychology*, 43(Pt 2): 225–44.

Dania, G., Vander Hoorn, S., Lopex, A.D., Murray, C.J. and Ezzati, M. (2005)

'Causes of cancer in the world: comparative risk assessment of nine behavioural and environmental risk factors', *Lancet*, 366(9499): 1784–93.

Davey Smith, G. (1996) 'Income inequality and mortality: why are they related? Income inequality goes hand in hand with under investment in human resources', *British Medical Journal*, 312: 987–8.

Davey Smith, G., Hart, C., Blane, D., Gillis, C. and Hawthorne, V. (1997) 'Lifetime socio-economic position and mortality: prospective observational study', *British Medical Journal*, 314: 547–52.

Davies, C. (1984) 'General practitioners and the pull of prevention', *Sociology of Health and Illness*, 6(3): 267–89.

Davis, A. and George, J. (1990) *States of Health: Health and Illness in Australia*, Sydney: Harper and Row.

Davison, C. and Davey Smith, G. (1995) 'The baby and the bath water: examining socio-cultural and free market critiques of health promotion', in R. Bunton, S. Nettleton and R. Burrows (1995) *The Sociology of Health Promotion*, Routledge: London.

Davison, C., Frankel, S. and Davey Smith, G. (1989) 'Inheriting heart trouble – the relevance of common-sense ideas to preventive measures', *Health Education Research – Theory and Practice*, 4: 329–40.

Davison, C., Smith, G. and Frankel, S. (1991) 'Lay epidemiology and the prevention paradox: the implications of coronary candidacy for health education', *Sociology of Health and Illness*, 13(1): 1–19.

Davison C., Frankel, S. and Smith, G. (1992) 'The limits of lifestyle: re-assessing "fatalism" in the popular culture of illness prevention', *Social Science and Medicine*, 34(6): 675–85.

Davison, C., Macintyre, S. and Smith, G. (1994) 'The potential social impact of predictive genetic testing for susceptibility to common chronic disease: a review and proposed research agenda', *Sociology of Health and Illness*, 16 (3): 340–71.

Davison, R., Hunt, K. and Kitzinger, J. (1999) ' "That could be down the road": lay perceptions of images of poverty and inequality', paper presented at 1999 Medical Sociology conference cited in J. Popay, S. Bennett, C. Thomas, G. Williams, A. Gatrell and L. Bostock, (2003) 'Beyond "beer, fags, eggs and chips"? Exploring lay understandings of social inequalities in health', *Sociology of Health and Illness*, 25(1): 1–23.

Dean, K. (1993) 'Integrating theory and methods in population health research', in K. Dean (ed.) *Population Health Research: Linking Theory and Methods*, London: Sage.

Dean, K., Concha, C. and Santiago, P.H. (1995) 'Research on lifestyles and health: searching for meaning', *Social Science and Medicine*, 41(6): 845–55.

Dean, M. (1999) *Governmentality: Power and Rule in Modern Society*, London: Sage.

Dedman, D.J., Gunnell, D., Davey Smith, G. and Frankel, S. (2001) 'Childhood housing conditions and later mortality in the Boyd Orr cohort', *Journal of Epidemiology and Community Health*, 55: 10–15.

Denton, M., Prus, S. and Walters, V. (2004) 'Gender differences in health: a Canadian study of the psychosocial, structural and behavioural determinants of health', *Social Science and Medicine*, 58: 2585–600.

Denzin, N. and Lincoln, Y. (1994) *Handbook of Qualitative Research*, Thousand Oaks, Calif.: Sage.

Dey, I. (1993) *Qualitative Data Analysis: a User Friendly Guide for Social Scientists*, London: Routledge.

Dines, A. and Cribb, A. (eds) (1993) *Health Promotion, Concepts and Practice*, Oxford: Blackwell Scientific Publications.

Dingwall, R. (1976) *Aspects of Illness*, London: Martin Robertson.

Donahue, J. and McGuire, M. (1995) 'The political economy of responsibility in health and illness', *Social Science and Medicine*, 4(1): 47–53.

Douglas, M. (1990) 'Risk as a forensic resource', *Daedalus*, 19(4): 1–16.

Douglas, M. (1992) *Risk and Blame: Essays in Cultural Theory*, New York: Routledge.

Dozier, S., Wagner, R.F. Jr, Black, S.A. and Terracina, J. (1997) 'Beachfront screening for skin cancer in Texas gulf coast surfers', *Southern Medical Journal*, 90(1): 55–8.

Duff, J. (1999) 'Dietary guidelines, corporate interests, and nutrition policy', in J. Germov and L. Williams (eds) *A Sociology of Food and Nutrition: the Social Appetite*, Melbourne: Oxford University Press.

Easthope, G. (1993) 'The response of orthodox medicine to the challenge of alternative medicine in Australia', *The Australian and New Zealand Journal of Sociology*, 29(3): 289–301.

Easthope, G. (2004) 'Consuming health: the market for complementary and alternative medicine', *Australian Journal of Primary Health*, 10(2): 68–75.

Easthope, G., Tranter, B. and Gill, G. (2000a) 'General practitioners' attitudes toward complementary therapies', *Social Science and Medicine*, 51(10): 1555–61.

Easthope, G., Tranter, B. and Gill, G. (2000b) 'The normal medical practice of referring patients for complementary therapies among Australian general practitioners', *Journal of Complementary Therapies in Medicine*, 8(4): 226–33.

Easthope, G., Beilby, J., Gill, G. and Tranter, B. (1998) 'Acupuncture in Australian general practice: practitioner characteristics', *Medical Journal of Australia*, 169(4): 197–200.

Eastwood, H. (2000) 'Complementary therapies: the appeal to general practitioners', *Medical Journal of Australia*, 173: 95–8.

Ebrahim, S. and Davey Smith, G. (1997) 'Systematic review of randomised controlled trials of multiple risk factor interventions for preventing coronary disease', *British Medical Journal*, 314: 1666.

Ebrahim, S. and Davey Smith, G. (2000) 'Multiple risk factor interventions for primary prevention of coronary heart disease', *Cochrane Data Base Systematic Review*, 2000(2): CD001561.

Ebrahim, S., Smith, G.D. and Bennett, R. (2000) 'Health promotion activity should be retargeted at secondary prevention', *British Medical Journal*, 320: 185.

Edmunds, L., Waters, E. and Elliot, E.J. (2001) 'Evidence based management of childhood obesity', *British Medical Journal*, 323: 916–19.

Egger, G., Donovan, R. and Spark, R. (1993) *Health and the Media: Principles and Practices for Health Promotion*, Sydney: McGraw-Hill Book Company.

Ehrenreich, B. and English, D. (1974) *Complaints and Disorders: the Sexual Politics of Sickness*, London: Compendium.

Elley, C.R., Kerse, N., Arroll, B. and Robinson, E. (2003) 'Effectiveness of counselling patients on physical activity in general practice: cluster randomised controlled trial', *British Medical Journal*, 327: 498–500.

Elstein, A.S. (1976) 'Clinical judgement, psychological research and medical practice', *Science*, 194: 696–700.

Emslie, C., Hunt, K. and Watt, G. (2001) 'Invisible women? Gender, lay beliefs and heart problems', *Sociology of Health and Illness*, 23(2): 203–33.

Engel, G.L. (1981) 'The need for a new medical model: a challenge for bio-medicine', in A.I. Caplan, H.T. Engelhardt Jr and J.J. Macartney (eds) *Concepts of Health and Disease: Interdisciplinary Perspectives*, Reading Mass.: Addison Wesley.

Epstein, J. (1995) *Altered Conditions: Disease, Medicine and Storytelling*, New York: Routledge.

Epstein, S.S. (1978) *The Politics of Cancer*, San Francisco: Sierra Club Books.

Epstein, S.S. (1990) 'Losing the war against cancer: who's to blame and what to do about it', *International Journal of Health Services*, 20(1): 53–71.

Evans, R.J. (1992) 'Epidemics and revolutions: cholera in nineteenth century Europe', in T. Ranger and P. Slack (eds) *Epidemics and Ideas: Essays on the Historical Perception of Pestilence*, Cambridge: Cambridge University Press.

Eyles, J., Brimblecombe, M., Chaulk, P., Stoddart, G., Pranger, T. and Moase, O. (2001) 'What determines health? To where should we shift resources? Attitudes towards the determinants of health among multiple stakeholder groups in Prince Edward Island, Canada', *Social Science and Medicine*, 53(2001): 1611–19.

Faber, M. and Rheinhardt, A. (1982) *Promoting Health through Risk Reduction*, New York: Macmillan.

Fabrega, H. (1974) *Disease and Social Behaviour*, Cambridge, Mass.: MIT Press.

Featherstone, M. (1987) 'Lifestyle and consumer culture', *Theory, Culture and Society*, 4(1): 55–70.

Featherstone, M. (1991) *Consumer Culture and Postmodernism*, London: Sage.

Featherstone, M., Hepworth, M. and Turner, B.S. (eds) (1991) *The Body: Social Process and Cultural Theory*, London: Sage.

Feinstein, A.R. (1985) *Clinical Epidemiology*, Philadelphia, Pa.: Saunders.

Fitzgerald, F.T. (1994) 'The tyranny of health', *New England Journal of Medicine*, 331(31): 196–9.

Fitzpatrick, M. (2001) *The Tyranny of Health: Doctors and the Regulation of Lifestyle*, Routledge: London.

Fleck, L. (1979) *Genesis and Development of a Scientific Fact*, ed. T.J. Trenn and R.K. Merton, trans. F. Bradley and T.J. Trenn, Chicago: The University of Chicago Press.

Flick, U. (1998) 'The social construction of individual and public health: contributions of social representations theory to a social science of health', *Social Science Information*, 37(4): 639–62.

Florin, D. (1999) 'Scientific uncertainty and the role of expert advice: the case of health checks for coronary heart disease prevention by general practitioners in the UK', *Social Science and Medicine*, 49(1999): 1269–83.

Førde, O.H. (1998) 'Is imposing risk awareness cultural imperialism?', *Social Science and Medicine*, 47(9): 1155–9.

Foster, G. and Anderson, B. (1978) *Medical Anthropology*, New York: John Wiley.

Foster, P. (1995) *Women and the Health Care Industry: an Unhealthy Relationship?*, Buckingham: Open University Press.

Fox, N.J. (1992) *The Social Meaning of Surgery*, Milton Keynes: Open University Press.

Fox, N.J. (1993) *Postmodernism, Sociology and Health*, Buckingham: Open University Press.

Fox, N.J. (1999) *Beyond Health: Postmodernism and Embodiment*, London: Free Association Books.

Fox, P. (1989) 'From senility to Alzheimer's disease: the rise of the Alzheimer's disease movement', *Millbank Quarterly*, 67(1): 58–102.

Fox, R. (1977) 'The medicalization and demedicalization of American society', *Daedalus*, 106(1): 9–22.

Fox, R. (2000) 'Medical uncertainty revisited', in G.L. Albrecht, R. Fitzpatrick and S.C. Scrimshaw (eds) *Handbook of Social Studies in Health and Medicine*, London: Sage Publications.

Frank, A.W. (1997) 'Blurred inscriptions of health and illness', *Body and Society*, 3(2): 103–13.

Frankel, S., Davison, C. and Smith, G.D. (1991) 'Lay epidemiology and the rationality of responses to health education', *British Journal of General Practice*, 41(351): 428–30.

Freidson, E. (1970) *Profession of Medicine*, New York: Dodd-Mead.

French, D.P., Maissi, E. and Marteau, T.M. (2005) 'The purpose of attributing cause: beliefs about the causes of myocardial infarction', *Social Science and Medicine*, 60: 1411–21.

French, R. (1994) 'Triumph over multiple sclerosis', *Australian Wellbeing Magazine*, 56 (July): 102.

Freund, P. and McGuire, M. (1991) *Health, Illness and the Social Body: a Critical Sociology*, Paramus, NJ: Prentice Hall.

Fullagar, S. (2002) 'Governing the healthy body: discourses of leisure and lifestyle within Australian health policy', *Health*, 6(1): 69–84.

Fulton, J.E., McGuire, M.T., Caspersen, C.J. and Dietz, W.H. (2001) 'Interventions for weight loss and weight gain prevention among youth: current issues', *Sports Medicine*, 31(3): 153–65.

Furner, V. and Ross, M. (1993) 'Lifestyle clues in the recognition of HIV infection: how to take a sexual history', *Medical Journal of Australia*, 158(1): 40–1.

Furnham, A.F. (1988) *Lay Theories: Everyday Understanding of Problems in the Social Sciences*, Oxford: Pergamon.

Fylkesnes, K. and Førde, O. (1993a) 'Determinants and dimensions involved in self-evaluation of health', *Social Science and Medicine*, 35: 271–9.

Fylkesnes, K. and Førde, O. (1993b) 'Determinants of health care utilization. Visits and referrals', *Scandinavian Journal of Social Medicine*, 21: 40–50.

Gabbay, J. (1982) 'Asthma attacked? Tactics for the reconstruction of a disease concept', in P. Wright and A. Treacher (eds) *The Problem of Medical Knowledge: Examining the Social Construction of Medicine*, Edinburgh: Edinburgh University Press.

Gabe, J., Calnan, M. and Bury, M. (eds) (1991) *The Sociology of Health Service*, London: Routledge.

Gaines, A.D. and Hahn, R.A. (1985) 'Among the physicians: encounter, exchange, and transformation', in R.A. Hahn and A.D. Gaines (eds) *Physicians of Western Medicine: Anthropological Approaches to Theory and Practice*, Dordrecht: Reidel Publishing Company.

Gammon, D.A. (1990) *Patients and Methods: Clinical Methods Applied to General Practice*, Sydney: McGraw-Hill Book Company.

Germov, J. (1997) 'Class, health inequality and social justice', in J. Germov (ed.) *Second Opinion: an Introduction to Health Sociology*, Melbourne: Oxford University Press.

Germov, J. (ed.) (2004) *Second Opinion: an Introduction to Health Sociology*, 3rd edn, Melbourne: Oxford University Press.

Germov, J. and Williams, L. (eds) (1999) *A Sociology of Food and Nutrition: the Social Appetite*, Melbourne: Oxford University Press.

Gerson, M., Grega, C.H. and Berger, S.J. (1993) 'Three kinds of coping: families and inflammatory bowel disease', *Family Systems Medicine*, 11(1): 55–65.

Getz, L., Sigurdsson, J. and Hetlevik, I. (2003) 'Is opportunistic disease prevention in the consultation ethically justifiable?', *British Medical Journal*, 327: 498–500.

Giard, R.W. (2003) 'Screening: careful considerations versus commercial medicine', *Ned Tijdschr Geneeskd*, 14(39): 1893–6.

Giddens, A. (1991) *Modernity and Self Identity: Self and Society in the Late Modern Age*, Oxford: Polity Press.

Glassner, B. (1989) 'Fitness and the postmodern self', *Journal of Health and Social Behaviour*, 30(2): 180–91.

Golan, M. and Weizman, A. (2001) 'A familial approach to the treatment of childhood obesity: a conceptual model', *Journal of Nutrition Education*, 33(2): 102–7.

Goldstein, M. (1992) *The Health Movement: Promoting Fitness in America*, New York: Twayne Publishing.

Goldstein, M.S. (2000) 'The culture of fitness and the growth of CAM', in M. Kelner and B. Welman (eds) *Complementary and Alternative Medicine: Challenge and Change*, Amsterdam: Harwood Academic Publishers.

Good, B.J. (1994) *Medicine, Rationality and Experience: an Anthropological Perspective*, Cambridge: Cambridge University Press.

Good, B.J. and Good, M.J. (1980) 'The meaning of symptoms: a cultural hermeneutic model for clinical practice', in L. Eisenberg and A. Kleinman (eds) *The Relevance of Social Science for Medicine*, Dordrecht: Reidel Publishing Company.

Gordis, L. (1996) *Epidemiology*, New York: W.B. Saunders.

Gordon, D. (1988a) 'Tenacious assumptions in western medicine', in M. Lock and D. Gordon (eds) *Biomedicine Examined*, Dordrecht: Kluwer Academic Publishers.

Gordon, D. (1988b) 'Clinical science and clinical expertise: changing boundaries between art and science in medicine', in M. Lock and D. Gordon (eds) *Biomedicine Examined*, Dordrecht: Kluwer Academic Publishers.

Graham, H. (2002) 'Building an inter-disciplinary science of health inequalities: the example of lifecourse research', *Social Science and Medicine*, 55: 2005–16.

Grbich, C. (ed.) (1999) *Health in Australia: Sociological Concepts and Issues*, 2nd edn, Sydney: Prentice Hall Australia.

Greco, M. (1993) 'Psychosomatic subjects and the "duty to be well": personal agency within medical rationality', *Economy and Society*, 22(3): 357–72.

Green J. (1997) 'Risk and the construction of social identity: children's talk about accidents', *Sociology of Health and Illness*, 19(4): 457–79.

Grimshaw, J.M., Freemantle, N. and Wallace, S. (1995) 'Developing and implementing clinical practice guidelines', *Qualitative Health Care*, 4: 55–64.

Grundy, S.M., Pasternack, R., Greenland, P., Smith, S. and Fuster, V. (1999) 'Assessment of cardiovascular risk by use of multiple-risk-factor assessment equations: a statement for healthcare professionals from the American Heart association and the American College of Cardiology', downloaded 12 January 2006 from http://www.acc.org/clinical/consensus/risk/risk1.htm.

Guadagnoli, E. and Ward, P. (1998) 'Patient participation in decision making', *Social Science and Medicine*, 47(3): 329–39.

Gusfield, J.R. (1981) *The Culture of Public Problems*, Chicago: University of Chicago Press.

Hahn, R.A. (1983) 'Rethinking "illness" and "disease" ', in E.V. Daniel and J. Pugh (eds) *South Asian Systems of Healing; Special Volume: Contributions to Asian Studies XVIII*, Leiden: Brill.

Hale, C.N., Barker, D.J.P., Clark, P.M., Cox, L.J., Fall, C., Osmond, C. *et al.* (1991) 'Fetal and infant growth and impaired glucose tolerance at age 64', *British Medical Journal*, 303: 1019–22.

Hamilton, M., Waddington, P., Gregory, S. and Walker, A. (1995) 'Eat, drink and be saved: the spiritual significance of alternative diets', *Social Compass*, 42(4): 497–511.

Hansen, E. (2003a) 'Doctors as lay epidemiologists: areas of commonality between medical and lay accounts of lifestyle', paper in *Conference Proceedings of the Australian Sociological Association Conference*, University of New England, December 2003.

Hansen, E. (2003b) 'Patient explanatory models of chronic obstructive pulmonary disease (COPD)', Royal Australian College of General Practitioners Scientific Convention, 9 October, Hotel Grand Chancellor, Hobart.

Hansen, E. (2006) *Successful Qualitative Health Research: a Practical Introduction*, St Leonards, NSW: Allen and Unwin.

Hansen, E. and Walters J. (2004) 'How patients with chronic obstructive pulmonary disease (COPD) talk about their COPD and their perceptions of the relationship between cigarette smoking and developing COPD. Implications for smoking cessation counselling', Royal Australian College of General Practitioners 47th Annual Scientific Convention, Grand Hyatt Hotel, 30 September–3 October.

Harding, S. (1991) *Whose Science? Whose Knowledge? Thinking From Women's Lives*, New York: Cornell University Press.

Harvey, D. (1998) 'The body as an accumulation strategy', *Environment and Planning D – Society and Space*, 16(4): 410–21.

Hasler, J. and Schofield, T. (eds) (1984) *Continuing Care: the Management of Chronic Disease*, Oxford General Practice Series 7, Melbourne: Oxford Medical Publications.

Helman, C.G. (1978) 'Feed a cold, starve a fever – folk models of infection in an English suburban community and their relation to medical treatment', *Culture, Medicine and Psychiatry*, 2(2): 107–37.

Helman, C.G. (1981a) 'Disease versus illness in general practice', *Journal of the Royal College of General Practitioners*, 31(230): 548–52.

Helman, C.G. (1981b) 'Practice and planning: observations from general practice', *Social Science and Medicine*, 15(3): 415–19.

Helman, C.G. (1985a) 'Disease and pseudo-disease: a case history of pseudo-angina', in R.A. Hahn and A.D. Gaines (eds) *Physicians of Western Medicine: Anthropological Approaches to Theory and Practice*, Dordrecht: Reidel Publishing Company.

Helman, C.G. (1985b) 'Communication in primary care: the role of patient and practitioner explanatory models', *Social Science and Medicine*, 20(9): 923–31.

Helman, C.G. (1988) 'Psyche, soma and society: the social construction of psycho-somatic disorders', in M. Lock and D. Gordon (eds) *Biomedicine Examined*, Dordrecht: Kluwer Academic Publishers.

Henderson, B.J. and Maguire, B.T. (2000) 'Three lay mental models of disease inheritance', *Social Science and Medicine*, 50: 293–301.

Herzlich, C. and Pierret, J. (1987) *Illness and Self in Society*, Baltimore, Md.: John Hopkins University Press.

Heslop, P., Smith, G.D., Macleod, J. and Hart, C. (2001) 'The socioeconomic position of employed women, risk factors and mortality', *Social Science and Medicine*, 53(4): 477–85.

Hesse, M. (1963) *Models and Analogies in Science*, London: Routledge.

Hetzel, B. and McMichael, T. (1987) *The LS Factor: Lifestyle and Health*, Ringwood: Penguin Books Australia.

Heyman, B. (1998) 'Introduction' in B. Heyman (ed.) *Risk, Health and Health Care: a Qualitative Approach*, London: Arnold.

Heyman, B. and Henriksen, M. (1998) 'Values and health risks', in B. Heyman (ed.) *Risk, Health and Health Care: a Qualitative Approach*, London: Arnold.

Higginbotham, N., Heading, G., McElduff, P., Dobson, A. and Heller, R. (1999) 'Reducing coronary heart disease in the Australian coalfields: evaluation of a 10-year community intervention', *Social Science and Medicine*, 48(5): 683–92.

Hodgkin, K. (1978) *Towards Earlier Diagnosis in Primary Care*, 4th edn, New York: Churchill Livingstone.

Hoffmans, M.D.A.F., Kromhout, D. and de Lezenne Coulander, C. (1988) 'The impact of body mass index of 78,612 18 year old Dutch men on 32 year mortality from all causes', *Journal of Clinical Epidemiology*, 41: 749–56.

Holland, W.W. (ed.) (1970) *Data Handling in Epidemiology*, Oxford: Oxford University Press.

Holman, C.D. (1992) 'Something old, something new: perspectives on five "new" public health movements', *Health Promotion Journal of Australia*, 2(3): 4–11.

Hooper, L., Bartlett, C. Davey Smith, G. and Ebrahim, S. (2002) 'Systematic review of long term effects of advice to reduce dietary salt in adults', *British Medical Journal*, 325: 628.

Horton, M. and Aggleton, P. (1989) 'Perverts, inverts and experts: the cultural production of an AIDS research paradigm', in P. Aggleton, G. Hart and P. Davies (eds) *AIDS: Social Representations, Social Practices*, London: The Falmer Press.

Howlett, B.C., Ahmad, W.I.U. and Murray, R. (1992) 'An exploration of White, Asian and Afro-Caribbean peoples' concepts of health and illness causation', *New Community*, 18: 282–92.

Huang, B., Rodrigues, B.L., Burchfield, C.M., Chypu, P.H., Curb, J.D. and Yano, K. (1996) 'Acculturation and prevalence of diabetes among Japanese-American men in Hawaii', *American Journal of Epidemiology*, 144(7): 674–81.

Hubbard, R. and Wald, E. (1993) *Exploding the Gene Myth*, Boston, Mass.: Beacon Press.

Hughes, M. (1994) 'The risks of lifestyle and the diseases of civilisation', *Annual Review of Health Social Sciences*, 4: 57–78.

Hulley, S., Walsch, J. and Newman, T. (1992) 'Health policy on blood cholesterol: time to change directions', *Circulation*, 86(3): 1026–29.

Hume-Hall, R. (1990) *Health and the Global Environment*, Cambridge: Polity Press.

Huxley, R.R., Shiell, A.W. and Law, C.M. (2000) 'The role of size at birth and postnatal catch-up growth in determining systolic blood pressure: a systematic review of the literature', *Journal of Hypertension*, 18: 815–31.

Illich, I. (1979) *Limits to Medicine – Medical Nemesis: the Expropriation of Health*, Harmondsworth: Penguin.

Imperial Cancer Research Fund OXCHECK Study Group (1995) 'Effectiveness of health checks conducted by nurses in primary care: final results of the OXCHECK study', *British Medical Journal*, 310: 1099–104.

Inglis, B. and West, R. (1983) *The Alternative Health Guide*, London: Michael Joseph.

Iribarren, C., Jacobs, D.R., Kiefe, C.I., Lewis, C.E., Matthews, K.A., Roseman, J.M. and Hulley, S.B. (2005) 'Causes and demographic, medical, lifestyle and psychosocial predictors of premature mortality: the CARDIA study', *Social Science and Medicine*, 60(3): 471–82.

Irvine, R. (1999) 'Losing patients: health care, consumers, power and sociocultural change', in C. Grbich (ed.) *Health in Australia: Sociological Concepts and Issues*, 2nd edn, Sydney: Prentice Hall.

Jackson, C.L. (1992) 'Lifestyle counselling in general practice: waste of time or a challenge of skill?', *Medical Journal of Australia*, 157(6): 396–8.

Jackson, M. (1989) *Paths Toward a Clearing, Radical Empiricism and Ethnographic Inquiry*, Bloomington: Indiana University Press.

Jacobs, A.D., Ammerman, A.S., Ennett, S.T., Campbell, M.K., Tawney, K.W., Aytur, S.A., Marshall, S.W., Will, J.C. and Rosamond, W.D. (2004) 'Effects of a tailored follow-up intervention on health behaviours, beliefs, and attitudes', *Journal of Women's Health*, 13(5): 557–68.

Jacobs, D., Blackburn, H., Higgins, M., Reed, D., Iso, H., McMillan, G., Neaton, J., Nelson, J., Potter, J., Rifkind, B., Rossou, J., Shekelle, R. and Yusof, S. (1992) 'Report of the conference on low blood cholesterol: mortality associations', *Circulation*, 86(3): 1046–60.

Jaen, C., Stange, K. and Nutting, P. (1994) 'Competing demands of primary care: a model for the delivery of clinical preventive services', *Journal of Family Practitioners*, 38(2): 166–71.

Jefferis, B., Power, C., Graham, H. and Manor, O. (2004) 'Changing social gradients in cigarette smoking and cessation over two decades of adult follow-up in a British birth cohort', *Journal of Public Health*, 26(1): 13–18.

Johanson, M., Larsson, U.S., Säljö, R. and Svärdsudd, K. (1994) 'Lifestyle in primary healthcare discourse', *Social Science and Medicine*, 40(3): 339–48.

Johanson, M., Sätterlund, U., Larsson, U.S. and Svärdsudd, K. (1998) 'Lifestyle discussion in the provision of health care: an empirical study of patient–physician interaction', *Social Science and Medicine*, 47(1): 103–12.

Johnston, H.J., Jones, M., Riddler-Dutton, G., Spechler, F., Stokes, G.S. and Wyndham, L.E. (1995) 'Diet modification in lowering plasma cholesterol levels: a randomised trial of three types of intervention', *Medical Journal of Australia*, 162(10): 524–6.

Jonas, H.A., Dobson, A.J. and Brown, W.J. (2000) 'Patterns of alcohol consumption in young women', *The Australian and New Zealand Journal of Public Health*, 24(2): 185–91.

Julian, R. and Easthope, G. (1996) 'Migrant health', in C. Grbich (ed.) *Health in Australia: Sociological Concepts and Issues*, 2nd edn, Sydney: Prentice Hall Australia.

Kangas, I. (2002) ' "Lay" and "expert": illness knowledge constructions in the sociology of health and illness', *Health*, 6(3): 301–4.

Kaplan, R.M. (1988) 'The value dimension in studies of health promotion', in S. Spacapan and S. Oskamp (eds) *The Social Psychology of Health*, Newbury Park, Calif.: Sage.

Karasek, R. and Theorell, T. (1990) *Healthy Work: Stress, Productivity and the Reconstruction of Working Life*, New York: Basic Books.

Kavanagh, A. and Broom, D. (1998) 'Embodied risk: my body, myself?', *Social Science and Medicine*, 46(3): 437–44.

Kelaher, M., Paul, S., Lambert, H., Ahmad, W., Fenton, S. and Davey Smith, G. (2003) 'Ethnicity, health and health services utilization in a British study', *Critical Public Health*, 13(3): 229–31.

Keleher, H. (1994) 'Public health: challenges for nursing and allied health', in C. Waddell and A.R. Peterson (eds) *Just Health: Inequalities in Illness, Care and Prevention*, Melbourne: Churchill Livingstone.

Kelly, M. and Charlton, B. (1992) 'Health promotion: time for a new philosophy?', *British Journal of General Practice*, 42: 223–4.

Kelly, M. and Field, D. (1994) 'Comments on the rejection of the biomedical model in sociological discourse', *Medical Sociology News*, 19: 34–7.

Kelner, M. and Wellman, B. (2000) *Complementary and Alternative Medicine: Challenge and Change*, New York: Harwood Publishers.

Kemm, J.R. (2001) 'A birth cohort of smoking by adults in Great Britain 1974–1998', *Journal of Public Health Medicine*, 23(4): 306.

Kerr A., Cunningham-Burly, S. and Amos, A. (1998) 'The new genetics and health: mobilizing lay expertise', *Public Understanding of Science*, 7(1): 41–60.

Kickbusch, I. (1986a) 'Approaches to an ecological base for public health', *Health Promotion*, 4(4): 265–8.

Kickbusch, I. (1986b) 'Lifestyles and health', *Social Science and Medicine*, 22(2): 117–24.

Kirmayer, L. (1988) 'Mind and body as metaphors: hidden values in medicine', in M. Lock and D. Gordon (eds) *Biomedicine Examined*, Dordrecht: Kluwer Academic Publishers.

Kleiner, K. (1995) 'Why low cholesterol can get you down', *New Scientist*, 148(29): 10.

Kleinman, A. (1980) *Patients and Healers in the Context of Culture*, Berkeley: University of California Press.

Knafl, K.A. and Deatrick, J. A. (1986) 'How families manage chronic conditions: an analysis of the concept of normalisation', *Research in Nursing and Health*, 9(3): 215–22.

Knight, J. (1997) 'Models of health', in J. Germov (ed.) *Second Opinion: Sociology of Health and Illness*, Melbourne: Oxford University Press.

Kowal, E. and Paradies, Y. (2005) 'Ambivalent helpers and unhealthy choices: public health practitioners' narratives of indigenous ill-health', *Social Science and Medicine*, 60(6): 1347–57.

Kowalski, R.E. (1989) *The 8-Week Cholesterol Cure*, New York: Harper and Row.

Krieger, N. (1994) 'Epidemiology and the web of causation: has anyone seen the spider?', *Social Science and Medicine*, 39(7): 887–903.

Krug, G.J. (1995) 'Hepatitis C: discursive domains and epistemic chasms', *Journal of Contemporary Ethnography*, 24(3): 299–322.

Kuhn, T.S. (1970) *The Structure of Scientific Revolutions*, Chicago: University of Chicago Press.

Labonte, R. (1995) 'Population health and health promotion: what do they have to say to each other?', *Canadian Journal of Public Health*, 86(3): 165–8.

Laitakari, J., Miilunpalo, S. and Vuori, I. (1997) 'The process and methods of health counselling by primary health care personnel in Finland: a national survey', *Patient Education and Counselling*, 30(1): 61–70.

Lantz, P.M., House, J.S., Lepkowski, J.M., Williams, D.R., Mero, R.P. and Chen, J. (1998) 'Socioeconomic factors, health behaviours and mortality', *Journal of the American Medical Association*, 3279(21): 1703–46.

Last, J. (1988) *A Dictionary of Epidemiology*, 2nd edn, Oxford: Oxford University Press.

Launer, J. and Lindsey, C. (1997) 'Training for systemic general practice: a new approach from the Tavistock Clinic', *British Journal of General Practice*, 47(420): 453–6.

Lawler, D.A., Ebrahim, S. and Smith, G.D. (2002) 'Is there a sex difference in the association between birth weight and systolic blood pressure in later life? Findings from a meta-regression analysis', *American Journal of Epidemiology*, 156: 1100–4.

Lawler, D.A., Frankel, S., Ebrahim, S. and Davey Smith, G. (2003) 'Smoking and ill health: does lay epidemiology explain the failure of smoking cessation programs among deprived populations?', *American Journal of Public Health*, 93(2): 266–70.

Lawson, J. (1991) *Public Health Australia: an Introduction*, Sydney: McGraw Hill.

Lawton, J. (2002) 'Colonising the future: temporal perceptions and health-relevant behaviours across the adult lifecourse', *Sociology of Health and Illness*, 24(6): 714–33.

Layder, D. (1993) *New Strategies in Social Research: an Introduction and Guide*, Cambridge: Polity Press.

Le Fanu, J. (1986) 'Diet and disease: nonsense and non-science', in D. Anderson (ed.) *A Diet of Reason: Sense and Nonsense in the Healthy Eating Debate*, London: The Social Affairs Unit.

Le Fanu, J. (1999) *The Rise and Fall of Modern Medicine*, London: Little, Brown and Company.

Leichter, H.M. (2003) ' "Evil habits" and "personal choices": assigning responsibility for health in the 20th century', *Milbank Quarterly*, 81(4): 603–26.

Levine, A.G. (1982) *Love Canal: Science, Politics and People*, Lexington, Mass.: D.C. Heath.

Lewis, B. and Ridge, D.T. (2005) 'Mothers reframing physical activity: family oriented politicism, transgression and contested priorities in Australia', *Social Science and Medicine*, 60 (10): 2295–306.

Lewis, D.K. and Barton, S. (2003) 'Who decides when to start preventive treatment? A questionnaire survey to compare the views of different population subgroups', *Journal of Epidemiology and Community Health*, 57: 241–2.

Lewis, D.K., Robinson, J. and Wilkinson, E. (2003) 'Factors involved in deciding to start preventive treatment: qualitative study of clinicians' and lay people's attitudes', *British Medical Journal*, 327: 841–4.

Leyland, A.H. (2004) 'Increasing inequalities in premature mortality in Great Britain', *Journal of Epidemiology and Community Health*, 58(4): 296–302.

Lindenbaum, S. and Lock, M. (eds) (1993) *Knowledge, Power and Practice: the*

Anthropology of Medicine and Everyday Life, Berkeley: University of California Press.

Link, B. and Phelan, J. (1995) 'Social conditions as fundamental causes of disease', *Journal of Health and Social Behavior* (Extra Issue): 80–94.

Livesey, P. (1986) *Partners in Care: the Consultation in General Practice*, London: William Heinemann Medical Books.

Lock, M. (1985) 'Models and practice in medicine: menopause as a symptom or life transition', in R.A. Hahn and A.D. Gaines (eds) *Physicians of Western Medicine: Anthropological Approaches to Theory and Practice*, Dordrecht: D. Reidel.

Lock, M. (1986) 'Introduction: anthropological approaches to menopause: questioning received wisdom', *Culture, Medicine and Psychiatry*, 10(1): 1–5.

Lock, M. (1988) 'A nation at risk: interpretations of school refusal in Japan', in M. Lock and D. Gordon (eds) *Biomedicine Examined*, Dordrecht: Kluwer Academic Publishers.

Lock, M. and Gordon, D. (eds) (1988a) *Biomedicine Examined*, Dordrecht: Kluwer Academic Publishers.

Lock, M. and Gordon, D. (1988b) 'Relationships between society, culture and biomedicine: introduction to the essays', in M. Lock and D. Gordon (eds) *Biomedicine Examined*, Dordrecht: Kluwer Academic Publishers.

Lofland, J. and Lofland, L. (1984) *Analyzing Social Settings*, 2nd edn, Belmont, Calif.: Wadsworth.

Lomas, J. (1998) 'Social capital and health: implications for public health and epidemiology', *Social Science and Medicine*, 47(9): 1181–8.

Love, R., Jackson, L., Edwards, R. and Pederson, A. (1997) 'Gender and its relationship to other determinants of health', position paper, Fifth National Health Promotion Conference, Halifax, Nova Scotia: Department of Behavioural Science, University of Toronto.

Lowenberg, J.S. and Davis, F. (1994) 'Beyond medicalisation-demedicalisation: the case of holistic health', *Sociology of Health and Illness*, 16(5): 579–99.

Lucas, A., Fewtrell, M.S. and Cole, T.J. (1999) 'Fetal origin of adult disease – the hypothesis revisited', *British Medical Journal*, 319: 245–9.

Lunney, J. (1993) 'Development of a program of health promotion research', in J. Wilson-Barnett and J. Macleod-Clark (eds) *Research in Health Promotion and Nursing*, London: Macmillan.

Lupton, D. (1993) 'Risk as moral danger: the social and political functions of risk discourse in public health', *International Journal of Health Services*, 23(3): 425–35.

Lupton, D. (1994a) *Medicine as Culture: Illness, Disease and the Body in Western Societies*, London: Sage.

Lupton, D. (1994b) 'The great debate about cholesterol: medical controversy and the news media', *Australian and New Zealand Journal of Sociology*, 30(3): 334–9.

Lupton, D. (1995) *The Imperative of Health: Public Health and the Regulated Body*, London: Sage.

Lupton, D. (1997) 'Foucault and the medicalisation critique', in A. Peterson and R. Bunton (eds) *Foucault, Health and Medicine*, London: Routledge.

Lupton, D. (1999) 'Developing the "whole me": citizenship, neo-liberalism and the contemporary health and physical education curriculum', *Critical Public Health*, 9(4): 287–300.

Lupton, D. (2002) 'The body, medicine and society', in J. Germov (ed.) *Second*

Opinion: an Introduction of Health Sociology, 2nd edn, South Melbourne: Oxford University Press.

Lupton, D. (2004) ' "A grim health future": food risks in the Sydney press', *Health, Risk and Society*, 6(2): 187–200.

Lynch, J.W. and Davey Smith, G. (2002) 'Commentary: income inequality and health: the end of the story?', *International Journal of Epidemiology*, 31: 549–51.

Lynch, J.W., Davey Smith, G., Kaplan, G.A. and House, J.S. (2000) 'Income inequality and mortality: importance to health of individual income, psychosocial environment, or material conditions', *British Medical Journal*, 320: 1200–4.

Lynch, J.W., Davey Smith, G., Harper, S., Hillmeier, M., Ross, N., Kaplan, G.A. and Wolfson, M. (2004) 'Is income inequality a determinant of health? Part 1. A systematic review', *Milbank Quarterly*, 82(1): 5–99.

Macintyre, S., McKay, L. and Ellaway, A. (2005) 'Are rich people or poor people more likely to be ill? Lay perceptions, by social class and neighbourhood, of inequalities in health', *Social Science and Medicine*, 60: 313–17.

McKee, J. (1988) 'Holistic health and the critique of western medicine', *Social Science and Medicine*, 26(8): 775–84.

McKeigue, P. and Marmot, M. (1988) 'Mortality from coronary heart disease in London', *British Medical Journal*, 297: 903.

McKenna, J. and Vernon, M. (2004) 'How general practitioners promote "lifestyle" physical activity', *Patient Education and Counselling*, 54(1): 101–6.

Mackie, J., Groves, K., Hoyle, A., Garcia, C., Garcia, R., Gunson, B. and Neuberger, J. (2001) 'Orthopic liver transplantation for alcoholic liver disease: a retrospective analysis of survival, recidivism and risk factors predisposing to recidivism', *Liver Transplantation*, 7: 418–27.

McKinlay, E., Plumridge, L., McBain, L., McLeod, D., Pullon, S. and Brown, S. (2005) ' "What sort of health promotion are you talking about?" A discourse analysis of the talk of general practitioners', *Social Science and Medicine*, 60: 1099–106.

McKinlay, J.B. (1993) 'The promotion of health through planned sociopolitical change: challenges for research and policy', *Social Science and Medicine*, 36: 109–17.

McKinlay, J.B. (1994) 'Towards appropriate levels of analysis, research methods and health public policy', paper presented at the International Symposium on Quality of Life and Health: Theoretical and Methodological Considerations, 25–27 May, Berlin.

MacMahon, B. and Pugh, T.F. (1970) *Epidemiology: Principles and Methods*, Boston: Little, Brown and Company.

McPherson, P.D. (1992) 'Health for all Australians', in H. Gardner (ed.) *Health Policy*, Melbourne: Churchill Livingstone.

McWhinney, I.R. (1989) *A Textbook of Family Medicine*, New York: Oxford University Press.

Malinas, R.M. (2001) 'Physical activity and fitness: pathways from childhood to adulthood', *American Journal of Human Biology*, 13(2): 162–72.

Mant, D. (1989) 'Breast self-examination: should we discourage it?', *Journal of the Royal College of General Practitioners*, 39(322): 180–1.

Marang-van de Mheen, P.J., Smith, G.D. and Hart, C.L. (1999) 'The health impact of smoking in manual and non-manual social class men and women: a test of the Blaxter hypothesis', *Social Science and Medicine*, 48(12): 1851–6.

Marmot, M. and Wilkinson R.G. (eds) (1999) *Social Determinants of Health*, Oxford: Oxford University Press.

Marmot, M.G., Rose, G., Shipley, M. and Hamilton, P.J.S. (1978) 'Employment grade and coronary heart disease in British civil servants', *Journal of Epidemiology and Community Health*, 32(4): 244–9.

Marmot, M.G, Davey Smith, G., Stansfield, S., Patel, C., North, F., Head, J., White, L., Brunner, E. and Feeney, A. (1991) 'Health inequalities among British civil servants: the Whitehall II Study', *Lancet*, 337(8747): 1387–93.

Martin, E. (1987) *The Woman in the Body*, Milton Keynes: Open University Press.

Martin, E. (1990) 'Toward an anthropology of immunology: the body as nation state', *Medical Anthropology Quarterly*, 4(4): 410–26.

Martin, E. (1994) *Flexible Bodies: Tracking Immunity in American Culture – From the Days of Polio to the Age of AIDS*, Boston, Mass.: Beacon Press.

May, C. and Sirur, D. (1998) 'Art, science and placebo: incorporating homeopathy in general practice', *Sociology of Health and Illness*, 20(2): 168–90.

Mechanic, D. (1994) 'Promoting health: implications for modern and developing nations', in L. Chen, A. Kleinman and N. Ware (eds) *Health and Social Change in International Perspective*, Cambridge, Mass.: Harvard University Press.

Metagenics (1999) *Inner Cleansing: the Gut Repair and Liver Detoxification Program*, Health World Limited, Kingsford Smith Drive, Queensland, photo-copied and distributed by their agent Janice Dance, PO Box 90, Newtown, Hobart, Australia 7009.

Metcalfe, A. (1993) 'Living in a clinic: the power of public health promotions', *Australian Journal of Anthropology*, 4(1): 31–44.

Miles, M. and Huberman, A.M. (1994) *Qualitative Data Analysis*, Beverly Hills, Calif.: Sage.

Milner, J. (1998) 'Understanding postmodernism: "Cliffs Notes" for sociologists', conference paper presented at the American Sociological Association (ASA).

Milner, S. (1998) 'Reconceptualising risk in health-promotion practice', in B. Heyman (ed.) *Risk, Health and Health Care: a Qualitative Approach*, London: Arnold.

Misselbrook, D. and Armstrong, D. (2002) 'Thinking about risk. Can doctors and patients talk the same language?', *Family Practice*, 19(1): 1–2.

Monaem, A. (1989) 'An orientation to health promotion', in G.M. Lupton and J.M. Najman (eds) *Sociology of Health and Illness: Australian Readings*, Melbourne: Macmillan Australia.

Montgomery, S. (1991) 'Of codes and combat: images of disease in biomedical discourse', *Science as Culture*, 12: 55–73.

Montgomery, S. (1993) 'Illness and image in holistic discourse: how alternative is alternative?', *Cultural Critique*, 25: 65–89.

Morgan, D.L. (1997) *Focus Groups as Qualitative Research*, Newbury Park, Calif.: Sage.

Morrell, D. (1991) *The Art of General Practice*, London: Oxford Medical Publications; Oxford University Press.

Mostyn, B. (1985) 'The content analysis of qualitative research data: a dynamic approach', in M. Brenner, J. Brown and D. Canter (eds) *The Research Interview: Uses and Approaches*, London: Academic Press.

Mudge, P., Hansen, E. and Walters, J. (2005) 'How patients with chronic obstructive pulmonary disease (COPD) describe their understandings of the relationship between cigarette smoking and COPD', free paper presented at the World Organisation of Family Doctors Asian Pacific Regional Conference, Kyoto, Japan, 27–31 May.

Murtagh, J. (1994) *General Practice*, London: McGraw Hill.

Must, A., Jacques, P.F., Dallal, G.E., Bajema, C.J. and Dietz, W.H. (1992) 'Long-term morbidity and mortality of overweight adolescents: a follow-up of the Harvard Growth study of 1922–1935', *New England Journal of Medicine*, 327: 1350–5.

Mutaner, C. and Lynch, J. (1999) 'Income inequality, social cohesion, and class relations: a critique of Wilkinson's neo-Durkheimian research program', *International Journal of Health Services*, 29: 59–81.

Naidoo, J. and Wills, J. (1998) *Practising Health Promotion: Dilemmas and Challenges*, London: Bailliere Tindall and the Royal College of Nursing.

Namekata, T., Moore, D.E., Suzuki, K., Mori, M., Knopp, R.H., Marcovina, S.M., Perrin, E.B., Hughes, D.A., Hatano, S. and Hayashi, C. (1997) 'Biological and lifestyle factors, and lipid and lipoprotein levels among Japanese Americans in Seattle and Japanese men in Japan', *International Journal of Epidemiology*, 26(6): 1203–13.

Narayan, K. and Venkat, M. (1997) 'Diabetes mellitus in Native Americans: the problem and its implications', *Population Research and Policy Review*, 16(1–2): 169–92.

National Health and Medical Research Council (NHMRC) (1992) *Dietary Guidelines for Australians*, Canberra: AGPS.

National Health and Medical Research Council (NHMRC) (1997) *Dietary Guidelines for Children and Adolescents*, Canberra: AGPS.

Navarro, V. (1976) *Medicine under Capitalism*, New York: Prodist.

Navarro, V. (1986) *Crisis, Health and Medicine: a Social Critique*, London: Tavistock.

Neighbour, R. (1987) *The Inner Consultation: How to develop an Effective and Intuitive Consulting Style*, Lancaster: MTP Press.

Neittaanmaki, L., Gross, E.B., Virjo, I., Hyppola, H. and Kumpusalo, E. (1999) 'Personal values of male and female doctors: gender aspects', *Social Science and Medicine*, 48(4): 559–68.

Nettleton, S. (1992) *Power, Pain and Dentistry*, Buckingham: Open University Press.

Nettleton, S. (1995) *The Sociology of Health and Illness*, Cambridge: Polity Press.

Nettleton, S. and Bunton, R. (1995) 'Sociological critiques', in R. Bunton, S. Nettleton and R. Burrows (eds) *The Sociology of Health Promotion: Critical Analyses of Consumption, Lifestyle and Risk*, London: Routledge.

New Zealand Guidelines Group (2003) 'The assessment and management of cardiovascular risk: best practice evidence based guideline', downloaded 12 January 2006 from http://www.nzgg.org.nz/index.cfm?fuseaction=fuseaction_10& fusesubaction=docs&documentid=22.

NHMRC (National Health and Medical Research Council) (2004) Website describing the 2004 General Practice Clinical Research Program, http://www.nhmrc.gov. au/research/genprac.htm, accessed 15 June 2005.

Nicolson, M. and McLaughlin, C. (1987) 'Social constructionism and medical sociology: a reply to M. Bury', *Sociology of Health and Illness*, 9(2): 107–27.

NIH (National Institute of Health) Consensus development panel of physical activity and cardiovascular health (1996) *Journal of American Medical Association*, 276(3): 241–6.

Nutting, P.A. (1986) 'Health promotion in primary medical care: problems and potential', *Preventive Medicine*, 15(5): 537–48.

Nyman, K.C. (1996) *Successful Consulting: a Practical Introduction to Consulting Skills in General Practice*, Melbourne: Royal Australian College of General Practitioners.

Oakley, A. (1989) 'Smoking in pregnancy: smokescreen or risk factor? Towards a materialist analysis', *Sociology of Health and Illness*, 11(4): 311–35.

O'Brian, M. (1995) 'Health and lifestyle: a critical mess? Notes on the de-differentiation of health', in R. Bunton, S. Nettleton and R. Burrows (eds) *The Sociology of Health Promotion: Critical Analyses of Consumption: Lifestyle and Risk*, London: Routledge.

O'Connor, M.L. and Parker, E. (1995) *Health Promotion: Principles and Practice in The Australian Context*, St Leonards, NSW: Allen and Unwin.

Oldenburg, B., Owen, N., Graham-Clarke, P. and Gomel, M. (1992) 'Lifestyle change and cardiovascular disease: principles and practice', *Australian Family Physician*, 21(9): 1289–93.

Oliver, M.F. (1992) 'Doubts about preventing coronary heart disease', *British Medical Journal*, 304: 393–4.

Olsen, J. and Trichopoulos, D. (1992) *Teaching Epidemiology: What You Should Know and What You Could Do*, Oxford: Oxford Medical Publications.

Ong, K.K.L., Ahmed, M.L., Emmett, P.M., Preece, M.A., Dunger, D.B. and the Avon Longitudinal Study of Pregnancy and Childhood Study Team (2000) 'Association between postnatal catch-up growth and obesity in childhood: prospective cohort study', *British Medical Journal*, 320: 967–71.

Open University (1985) *Experiencing and Explaining Disease*, Milton Keynes: The Open University Press.

Ornish, D., Brown, S.E., Scherwitz, L.W., Billings, J.H., Armstrong, W.T., Ports, T.A., McLanahan, S.M., Kirkeide, R.L., Brand R.J. and Gould, K.L. (1990) 'Can lifestyle changes reduce coronary heart disease?', *Lancet*, 36 (July): 129–33.

Owen, N. and Bauman, A. (1992) 'The descriptive epidemiology of a sedentary lifestyle in adult Australians', *International Journal of Epidemiology*, 21(2): 305–10.

Palmer, G.R. and Short, S.D. (1994) *Health Care and Public Policy: an Australian Analysis*, 2nd edn, Melbourne: Macmillan Education Australia.

Patton, C. (1986) *Sex and Germs: the Politics of AIDS*, Montreal: Black Rose Books.

Pearce, N. (1996) 'Traditional epidemiology, modern epidemiology, and public health', *American Journal of Public Health*, 86(5): 678–83.

Pearson, T.A. (1989) 'Influences on CHD incidence and case fatality: medical management of risk factors', *International Journal of Epidemiology*, 18(3 supp. 1): s217-s22.

Pels, R., Bor, D. and Lawrence, R. (1989) 'Decision-making for introducing clinical preventive services', *Annual Review of Public Health*, 10: 363–83.

Pender, N.J., Walker, S.N., Frank-Stromborg, N. and Sechrist, K.R. (1990) *Health Promotion in the Workplace: Making a Difference*, Dekalb: Northern Illinois University.

Peretti-Watel, P. (2004) 'Effects of using the epidemiology paradigm for studying risk-taking behaviours', *Revue Française de Sociologies*, 45(1): 103–32.

Pescosolido, B.A. and Kronenfeld, J.J. (1995) 'Health, illness, and healing in an uncertain era: challenges from and for a medical sociology', *Journal of Health and Social Behaviour* (Supp. Issue): 5–33.

Peters, S., Stanley, I., Rose, M. and Salmon, P. (1998) 'Patients with medically unexplained symptoms: sources of patient's authority and implications for demands on medical care', *Social Science and Medicine*, 46(4–5): 559–65.

Petersen, A. (1996) 'Risk and the regulated self: the discourse of health promotion as politics of uncertainty', *Australian and New Zealand Journal of Sociology*, 32(1): 44–57.

Petersen, A. and Lupton, D. (1996) *The New Public Health: Health and Self in the Age of Risk*, St Leonards, NSW: Allen and Unwin.

Petosa, R. (1984) 'Wellness: an emerging opportunity for health education', *Health Education*, 15(6): 37–9.

Phelan, J.C., Bruce, G., Diez-Roux, A., Kawachie, I. and Levin, B. (2004) ' "Fundamental causes" of social inequalities in mortality: a test of the theory', *Journal of Health and Social Behaviour*, 45(3): 265–85.

Pickstone, J.V. (1992) 'Death, dirt and fever epidemics: rewriting the history of British "public health", 1780–1850', in T. Ranger and P. Slack (eds) *Epidemics and Ideas: Essays on the Historical Perception of Pestilence*, Cambridge: Cambridge University Press.

Pierret, J. (1993) 'Constructing discourses about health and their social determinants', in A. Radley (ed.) *Worlds of Illness: Biographical and Cultural Perspectives on Health and Disease*, London: Routledge.

Pierret, J. (2003) 'The illness experience: state of knowledge and perspectives for research', *Sociology of Health and Illness*, 25 (Silver Anniversary Issue): 4–22.

Pilch, J. (1981) *Wellness: Your Invitation to a Full Life*, Minneapolis, Minn.: Winston Press.

Pill, R. (1991) 'Issues in lifestyles and health: lay meanings of health and health behaviour', in B. Badura and I. Kickbusch (eds) *Health Promotion Research: Towards a New Social Epidemiology*, WHO Regional Publications European Series no. 37, Copenhagen: World Health Organization, Regional Office for Europe.

Pirotta M., Cohen, M.M., Kostirilos, V. and Farish, S.J. (2000) 'Complementary therapies: have they become accepted in general practice?', *Medical Journal of Australia*, 172: 105–9.

Plant, A.J. and Rushworth, R. L. (1998) ' "Death by proxy": ethics and classification in epidemiology', *Social Science and Medicine*, 47(9): 1147–53.

Polglase, A.L., McDermott, F.T. and Hughes, E.S. (1984) 'Ulcerative colitis and Crohns disease, what your patient wants to know', *Australian Family Physician*, 13(6): 422–4.

Popay, J., Williams, G., Thomas, C. and Gatrell, T. (1998) 'Theorising inequalities in health: the place of lay knowledge', *Sociology of Health and Illness*, 20(5): 619–44.

Popay, J., Bennett, S., Thomas, C., Williams, G., Gatrell, A. and Bostock, L. (2003) 'Beyond "beer, fags, eggs and chips"? Exploring lay understandings of social inequalities in health', *Sociology of Health and Illness*, 25(1): 1–23.

Porter, R. (1997) *The Greatest Benefit to Mankind: a Medical History of Humanity from Antiquity to the Present*, London: Harper Collins.

Potts, L.K. (2004) 'An epidemiology of women's lives: the environmental risk of breast cancer', *Critical Public Health*, 14(2): 133–47.

Power, C. (1997) 'Measurement and long term health risks of childhood and adolescent fatness', *International Journal of Obesity*, 21: 507–26.

Prior, L. (2003) 'Belief, knowledge and expertise: the emergence of the lay expert in medical sociology', *Sociology of Health and Illness*, 25 (Silver Anniversary Issue): 41–57.

Prior, L., Pang Lai, C. and See Beng, H. (2000) 'Views on illness and health from two Cantonese speaking communities', *Sociology of Health and Illness*, 22(6): 815–39.

Puska, P. (1985) 'The community-based strategy to prevent coronary heart disease: conclusions from the ten years of the North Karelia project', *Annual Review of Public Health*, 6: 147–93.

RACGP (Royal Australian College of General Practitioners) (1998) *Putting Prevention into Practice: a Guide for the Implementation of Prevention in the General Practice Setting*, 1st edn, Melbourne: RACGP.

RACGP (Royal Australian College of General Practitioners) (2004) SNAP Guidelines downloaded from www.racgp.org.au, 19 May 2005.

Radley, A. (ed.) (1993) *Worlds of Illness: Biographical and Cultural Perspectives on Health and Disease*, London and New York: Routledge.

Remennick, L. (1998) 'Race, class, and occupation as determinants of cancer risk and survival: trend report: the cancer problem in the context of modernity: sociology, demography, politics', *Current Sociology*, 46(1): 25–39.

Rice, P.L. and Ezzy, D. (1999) *Qualitative Research Methods: a Health Focus*, Melbourne: Oxford University Press.

Richards, H., Reid, M. and Watt, C. (2003) 'Victim-blaming revisited: a qualitative study of beliefs about illness causation, and responses to chest pain', *Family Practice*, 20(6): 711–16.

Richards, M.P.M. (1993) 'The new genetics: some issues for social scientists', *Sociology of Health and Illness*, 15(5): 567–86.

Richardson, A. (1991) 'Health promotion through self help: the contribution of self-help groups', in B. Badura and I. Kickbusch (eds) *Health Promotion Research: Towards a New Social Epidemiology*, WHO Regional Publications European Series no. 37, Copenhagen: World Health Organization, Regional office for Europe.

Richmond, K. (1997) 'Health-promotion dilemmas', in J. Germov (ed.) *Second Opinion: Sociology of Health and Illness*, Melbourne: Oxford University Press.

Richmond, K. (2002) 'Health-promotion dilemmas', in J. Germov (ed.) *Second Opinion: Sociology of Health and Illness*, 2nd edn, Melbourne: Oxford University Press.

Riley, J.C. (1987) *The Eighteenth-Century Campaign to Avoid Disease*, New York: St Martin's Press.

Ritchie, J., Herscovitch, F. and Norfor, J. (1994) 'Beliefs of blue collar workers regarding coronary risk behaviours', *Health Education Research*, 9: 95–103.

Robinson, C.A. (1993) 'Managing life with a chronic condition: the story of normalization', *Qualitative Health Research*, 3(1): 6–28.

Rodmell, S. and Watts, A. (1986) 'The politics of health education: problems and possibilities', in S. Rodmell and A. Watts (eds) *The Politics of Health Education: Raising the Issues*, London: Routledge and Kegan Paul.

Rogers, W.S., Veale, B. and Weller, D. (1999) *Linking General Practice with Population Health: Report on GPEP Projects Investigating Population Health in General Practice*, Adelaide: Department of General Practice, Flinders University of South Australia.

Rose, G. (1992) *The Strategy of Preventive Medicine*, New York: Oxford University Press.

Rosenfeld, I. (1986) *Modern Prevention: the New Medicine*, New York: Simon and Schuster.

Ross, M. (1994) 'AIDS and the new public health', in C. Waddell and A.R. Petersen (eds) *Just Health: Inequality in Illness Care and Prevention*, London: Churchill Livingstone.

Rothman, K.J. (1998) *Modern Epidemiology*, Philadelphia, Pa.: Lippincott, Williams and Wilkins Publishers.

Rothstein, W.G. (2003) *Public Health and the Risk Factor*, Rochester, NY: University of Rochester Press.

Russell, D.G. and Buisson, D.H. (1988) *Lifestyle Report*, Dunedin: Human Performances Associates.

Russell, M. and Dobson, A. (1994) 'Age specific mortality from cardiovascular disease and other causes (1969–1990)', *Australian Journal of Public Health*, 18(2): 160–4.

Rutten, A. (1995) 'The implementation of health promotion: a new structural perspective', *Social Science and Medicine*, 41(12): 1627–37.

Ryan, E.L. and Skinner, C.S. (1999) 'Risk beliefs and interest in counselling: focus-group interviews among first-degree relatives of breast cancer patients', *Journal of Cancer Education*, 14(2): 99–103.

Sabo, D. and Gordon, D.F. (eds) (1995) *Men's Health and Illness: Gender, Power and the Body*, Newbury Park, Calif.: Sage Publications.

Sackett, D.L. (2002) 'The arrogance of preventative medicine', *Canadian Medical Association Journal*, 167(4): 363–4.

Sackett, D.L. Richardson, W.S., Rosenberg, W. and Haynes, R.B. (1997) *Evidence Based Medicine: How to Practise and Teach EBM*, London: Churchill Livingstone.

Sackett, D.L., Rosenberg, W.M.C., Gray, J.A.M. *et al.* (1996) 'Evidence based medicine: what it is and what it isn't', *British Medical Journal*, 313: 169–71.

Saggers, S. and Grey, D. (1991) *Aboriginal Health and Society: the Traditional and Contemporary Aboriginal Struggle for Better Health*, Sydney: Allen and Unwin.

Salonstall, R. (1993) 'Healthy bodies, social bodies: men's and women's concepts and practices of health in everyday life', *Social Science and Medicine*, 36(1): 7–14.

Savage, R. and Armstrong, D. (1990) 'Effect of a general practitioner's consulting style on patients' satisfaction: a controlled study', *British Medical Journal*, 301: 968–70.

Savage, M., Barlow, J., Dickens, P. and Fielding, T. (1992) *Property, Bureaucracy and Culture: Middle Class Formation in Contemporary Britain*, London: Routledge.

Schafer, R. (1979) 'The self-concept factor in diet selection and quality', *Journal of Nutrition Education*, 11: 37–9.

Scheingold, L. (1988) 'Balint work in England: lessons for American family medicine', *Journal of Family Practice*, 26(3): 315–20.

Schilling, C. (1991) 'Educating the body: physical capital and the production of social inequalities', *Sociology*, 25(4): 653–72.

Schlicht, S.M., Gordon, J.R., Ball, J.R. and Christie, D.G. (1990) 'Suicide and related deaths in Victorian doctors', *Medical Journal of Australia*, 153(9): 518–21.

Schutz, A. (1967) *The Phenomenology of the Social World*, trans. G. Walsh and F. Lenhert, Chicago: North Western University Press.

Seidman, I. (1998) *Interviewing as Qualitative Research: A Guide for Researchers in Education and the Social Sciences*, New York: Teachers College Press.

Shapiro, J. (1990) 'Patterns of psychosocial performance in the doctor–patient encounter: a study of family practice residents', *Social Science and Medicine*, 31(9): 1035–41.

Sharpe, C. and Buchanan, N. (1995) 'Juvenile myoclonic epilepsy: diagnosis, management and outcome', *Medical Journal of Australia*, 162(3): 133–4.

Shaw, I. (2002) 'How lay are lay beliefs?', *Health*, 6(3): 287–99.

Shim, J.K. (2002) 'Understanding the routinised inclusion of race, socioeconomic status and sex in epidemiology: the utility of concepts from technoscience studies', *Sociology of Health and Illness*, 24(2): 129–50.

Shostak, S. (2003) 'Locating gene-environment interaction: at the intersections of genetics ands public health', *Social Science and Medicine*, 56(2003): 2327–42.

Shy, C.M. (1997) 'The failure of academic epidemiology: witnesses for the prosecution', *American Journal of Epidemiology*, 145(6): 479–87.

Siahpush, M. (1998) 'Postmodern values, dissatisfaction with conventional medicine and popularity of alternative therapies', *Journal of Sociology*, 34(1): 58–70.

Siegler, M. (1981) 'The doctor–patient encounter and its relationship to theories of health and disease', in A.L. Caplan, H.T. Engelhardt Jr and J.J. McCartney (eds) *Concepts of Health and Disease: Interdisciplinary Perspectives*, Reading, Mass.: Addison Wesley.

Silagy, C. and Haines, A. (eds) (1998) *Evidence Based Practice in Primary Care*, London: BMJ Books.

Simpson, C. (1993) 'A process of dying by default', *Australian Family Physician*, 22(7): 1279–83.

Singh, G.R. and Hoy, W.E. (2003) 'The association between birthweight and current blood pressure: a cross-sectional study in an Australian Aboriginal community', *Medical Journal of Australia*, 179: 532–5.

Singh, I. (2004) 'Doing their jobs: mothering with Ritalin in a culture of mother-blame', *Social Science and Medicine*, 59(6): 1193–205.

Skolbekken, J. (1995) 'The risk epidemic in medical journals', *Social Science and Medicine*, 40(3): 291–305.

Skolbekken, J.A. (1998) 'Communicating the risk reduction achieved by cholesterol reducing drugs', *British Medical Journal*, 316(7149): 1956–8.

Smith, M. (1998) 'Community based epidemiology: community involvement in defining social risk', *Journal of Health and Social Policy*, 9(4): 51–65.

Smith, R.C., Gardiner, J.C., Lyles, J.S., Johnson, M., Rost, K.M., Luo, Z., Goddeeris, J., Lein, C., Given, C.W. and Given, B. (2002) 'Minor acute illness: a preliminary report on the "worried well" ', *Journal of Family Practice*, 51: 24–9.

Sontag, S. (1978) *Illness as Metaphor*, New York: Farrar, Strauss and Giroux.

Sontag, S. (1989) *Illness as Metaphor/AIDS and its Metaphors*, New York: Anchor Publishing.

Southern Tasmanian Division of General Practice (1999) *Health Needs Assessment for the Southern Division of General Practice June 1999*, The Southern Division of General Practice, 206 New Town Road, New Town, Tasmania.

Stacey, M. (1988) *The Sociology of Health and Healing*, London: Unwin Hyman.

Stampfer, M.J., Hu, F.B., Manson, J.E., Rimm, E.B. and Willett, W.C. (2000) 'Primary prevention of coronary heart disease in women through diet and lifestyle', *New England Journal of Medicine*, 343(1): 16–22.

Starr, P. (1982) *The Social Transformation of American Medicine: the Rise of a Sovereign Profession and the Making of A vast Industry*, New York: Basic Books.

Steptoe, A., Doherty, S., Rink, E., Kerry, S., Kendrick, T. and Hilton S. (1999) 'Behavioural counselling in general practice for the promotion of healthy behaviour among adults at increased risk of coronary heart disease: randomised trial', *British Medical Journal*, 319: 943–7.

Stewart, M.A. (1995) 'Effective physician–patient communication and outcomes: a review', *Canadian Medical Association Journal*, 152(9): 1423–33.

Storer, J.H., Cychosz, C.M. and Anderson, D.F. (1997) 'Wellness behaviours, social identities and health promotion', *The American Journal of Health Behaviour*, 21(4): 260–8.

Stott, N. (1994) 'Screening for cardiovascular risk in general practice', *British Medical Journal*, 308: 285–6.

Stott, N., Kinnersley, P. and Rollnick, S. (1994) 'The limits to health promotion', *British Medical Journal*, 309: 971–2.

Stott, N.C.H. (1986) 'The role of health promotion in primary medical care', *Health Promotion*, 1(1): 49–53.

Stott, N.C.H. and Pill, R.M. (1990) ' "Advice yes, dictate no". Patients' views on health promotion in the consultation', *Family Practice*, 7(2): 125–31.

Strandberg, M.D., Timo, E., Salomaa, M.D., Veikko, V. *et al.* (1991) 'Long-term mortality after 5-year multifactorial primary prevention of cardiovascular disease in middle-aged men', *Journal of the American Medical Association*, 266(9): 1225–9.

Strauss, A. and Corbin, J. (1994) 'Grounded theory methodology: an overview', in N.K. Denzin and Y.S. Lincoln (eds) *Handbook of Qualitative Research*, Seven Oaks: Sage.

Strauss, A. and Corbin, J. (1998) 'Grounded theory methodology: an overview', in N.K. Denzin and Y.S. Lincoln (eds) *Handbook of Qualitative Research*, 2nd edn, Sevenoaks: Sage.

Strong, P.M. (1979a) 'Sociological imperialism and the profession of medicine: a critical examination of the thesis of medical imperialism', *Social Science and Medicine*, 13A(2): 199–215.

Strong, P.M. (1979b) *The Ceremonial Order of the Clinic: Parents, Doctors and Medical Bureaucracies*, London: Routledge Kegan Paul.

Strong, P.M. (1984) 'Viewpoint: the academic encirclement of medicine?', *Sociology of Health and Illness*, 6(3): 339–58.

Susser, M. (1973) *Causal Thinking in the Health Sciences: Concepts and Strategies of Epidemiology*, London: Oxford University Press.

Susser, M. (1996) 'Choosing a future in epidemiology: eras and paradigms', *American Journal of Public Health*, 86(5): 668–73.

Swinford, P.A. and Webster, J. A. (1989) *Promoting Wellness: A Nurses' Handbook*, Rockville Md.: Aspen Publication.

Syme, S.L. (1996) 'To prevent disease: the need for a new approach', in D. Blane, E. Brunner and R. Wilkinson (eds) *Health and Social Organisation*, London: Routledge.

Synott, A. (1992) 'Tomb, temple, machine and self: the social construction of the body', *British Journal of Sociology*, 43(1): 79–110.

Synott A. (1993) *The Body Social: Symbolism, Self and Society*, London: Routledge.

Talley, N. and O'Connor, S. (1996) *Clinical Examination: a Systematic Guide to Physical Diagnosis*, 3rd edn, New York: MacLennan and Petty.

Tannahill, A. (1992) 'Epidemiology and health promotion: a common understanding', in R. Bunton and G. Macdonald (eds) *Health Promotion: Disciplines and Diversity*, London: Routledge.

Tapper-Jones, L.M. (1986) *Attitudes to Health Education Materials in General Practice*, Cardiff: University of Wales College of Medicine.

Tarlov, A.R. (2000) 'Coburn's thesis: plausible but we need more evidence and better measures', *Social Science and Medicine*, 51(2000): 993–5.

Taylor, R. and Ford, G. (1981) 'Lifestyle and aging: three traditions in lifestyle research', *Aging and Society*, 1(3): 329–45.

Temkin, O. (1981) 'The scientific approach to disease: specific entity and individual sickness', in A.L. Caplan, H.T. Englehardt Jr, and J.J. McCartney (eds) *Concepts of Health and Disease: Interdisciplinary Perspectives*, Reading, Mass.: Addison Wesley.

Terris, M. (1987) 'Epidemiology and the public health movement', *Journal of Public Health Policy*, 8(3): 315.

Terris, M. (1996) 'The development and prevention of cardiovascular disease risk factors: socioenvironmental influences', *Journal of Public Health Policy*, 17: 426–41.

Terris, M. (1998) 'Epidemiology and health policy in the Americas: meeting the neoliberal challenge', *Journal of Public Health Policy*, 19: 15–24.

Tesh, S.N. (1990) *Hidden Arguments: Political Ideology and Disease Prevention Policy*, New Brunswick: Rutgers University Press.

Thorne, S.E. (1993) *Negotiating Health Care: the Social Context of Chronic Illness*, Newbury Park, Calif.: Sage Publications.

Thouless, R.H. (1974) *Straight and Crooked Thinking*, London: Pan Books.

Toon, P.D. (1995) 'Health checks in general practice, time to review their role', *British Medical Journal*, 310: 1083–4.

Tuckett, D., Boulton, M., Olsen, C. and Williams, C. (1985) *Meetings Between Experts: an Approach to Sharing Ideas in Medical Consultations*, London: Tavistock.

Tudor-Smith, C., Nutbeam, D., Moore, L. and Catford, J. (1998) 'Effects of the Heartbeat Wales programme over five years on behavioural risks for cardiovascular disease: quasi-experimental comparison of results from Wales and matched reference areas', *British Medical Journal*, 316: 818–22.

Turner, B.S. (1987) *Medical Power and Social Knowledge*, London: Sage Publications.

Turner, B.S. (1991a) 'The discourse of diet', in M. Featherstone, M. Hepworth and B.S. Turner (eds) *The Body: Social Process and Cultural Theory*, London: Sage Publications.

Turner, B.S. (1991b) 'Recent developments in the theory of the body', in M. Featherstone, M. Hepworth and B.S. Turner (eds) *The Body: Social Process and Cultural Theory*, London: Sage.

Turner, B.S. (1996) *The Body and Society*, 2nd edn, London: Sage.

Twisk, J., Boreham, C., van Mechelen, W., Savage, M., Strain, J. and Cran, G. (1997) 'Relationships between the development of biological risk factors for coronary heart disease and lifestyle parameters during adolescence: the Northern Ireland Young Hearts project', *Public Health*, 113(1): 7–12.

University of Tasmania (1999) *1999 Course and Unit Handbook*, Hobart: University of Tasmania.

Usherwood, T. (1990) 'Responses to illness – implications for the clinician', *Journal of the Royal Society of Medicine*, 3(83): 205–7.

Usherwood, T. (1999) *Understanding the Consultation: Evidence, Theory and Practice*, Buckingham: Open University Press.

Van Beurden, E., James, R., Montague, D., Christian, J. and Dunn, T. (1993) 'Community-based cholesterol screening and education to prevent heart disease; five year results of the north coast cholesterol check campaign', *Australian Journal of Public Health*, 17: 109–16.

van Steenkiste, B., van der Weijden, T., Timmermans, D., Vaes, J., Stoffers, J. and Grol, R. (2004) 'Patients' ideas, fears and expectations of their coronary risk: barriers for primary prevention', *Patient Education and Counselling*, 55(2): 301–7.

Verbrugge, L.M. (1985) 'Gender and health: an update on hypotheses and evidence', *Journal of Health and Social Behaviour*, 26(3): 156–82.

Vertinsky, P. (1998) ' "Run Jane, Run": central tensions in the current debate about enhancing women's health through exercise', *Women and Health*, 27(4): 81–111.

Vigarello, G. (1988) *Concepts of Cleanliness: Changing Attitudes in France Since the Middle Ages*, trans. J. Birrell, Cambridge: Cambridge University Press.

Waddell, C. and Petersen, A.R. (eds.) (1994) *Just Health: Inequalities in Illness, Care and Prevention*, Melbourne: Churchill Livingstone.

Waldron, I. (1983) 'Sex differences in illness incidence, prognosis and mortality', *Social Science and Medicine*, 17: 1107–23.

Walsh, J. and McPhee, S. (1992) 'A systems model of clinical preventive care: an analysis of factors influencing patient and physician', *Health Education Quarterly*, 19(2): 157–75.

Walters, J., Hansen, E., Mudge, P., Johns, D., Walters, E.H. and Wood-Baker, R. (2005) 'Barriers to the use of spirometry in general practice for diagnosis and management of chronic obstructive pulmonary disease', *Australian Family Physician*, 34(3): 201–6.

Warde, A. (1994) 'Consumption, identity formation and uncertainty', *Sociology*, 28(4): 877–98.

Weatherall, D. (1995) *Science and the Quiet Art*, Oxford: Oxford University Press.

Weber, M. (1978) *Economy and Society*, vols I–II, trans. F.R. Guenther and C. Wittich, Berkeley: University of California Press.

Webster, A. (1991) *Science, Technology and Society*, London: Macmillan.

Welshman, J. (1996) 'Images of youth: the issue of juvenile smoking, 1880–1914', *Addiction*, 1(9): 1379–86.

West, P. (1979) 'An investigation in the social construction of consequences of the label epilepsy', *Sociological Review*, 27(4): 719–41.

White, K. (1994) 'Nineteenth century medicine, science, and values', in C. Waddell and A. Petersen (eds) *Just Health: Inequality in Illness, Care and Prevention*, Melbourne: Churchill Livingstone.

White, K. (2000) 'The state, the market and general practice: the Australian case', *International Journal of Health Services*, 30(2): 285–308.

White, K. (2002) *An Introduction to the Sociology of Health and Illness*, London: Sage Publications.

White, P., Young, K. and Gillett, J. (1995) 'Bodywork as a moral imperative: some critical notes on health and fitness', *Society and Leisure*, 18(1): 159–82.

Whittaker, A. (1995) 'Heart problems: coronary heart disease and risk in an

Australian suburb', paper presented at the Annual Public Health Association Conference, Cairns, Australia, 27–29 September.

Widgery, D. (1993) *Some Lives! A GP's East End*, London: Simon and Schuster.

Wiles, R. (1998) 'Patients' perceptions of their heart attack and recovery: the influence of epidemiological "evidence" and personal experience', *Social Science and Medicine*, 46(11): 1477–86.

Wilkie, T. (1994) *Perilous Knowledge: the Human Genome Project and Its Implications*, London: Faber and Faber.

Wilkinson, R.G. (1996) *Unhealthy Societies: the Afflictions of Inequality*, London: Routledge.

Wilkinson, R.G. (2000a) 'The need for an interdisciplinary perspective on the social determinants of health', *Health Economics*, 9: 581–3.

Wilkinson, R.G. (2000b) 'Deeper than "neoliberalism". A reply to David Coburn', *Social Science and Medicine*, 51(2000): 997–1000.

Wilkinson, R.G. (2004) 'The epidemiological transition: from material scarcity to social disadvantage', in M. Bury and J. Gabe (eds) *The Sociology of Health and Illness: a Reader*, London: Routledge.

Wilkinson, R.G. (2005) *The Impact of Inequality: How to Make Sick Societies Healthier*, New York: The New Press.

Willett, W. (1990) *Nutritional Epidemiology*, New York: Oxford University Press.

Williams, A. and Boulton, M. (1988) 'Thinking prevention: concepts and constructs in general practice', in M. Lock and D.R. Gordon (eds) *Biomedicine Examined*, Dordrecht: Kluwer Publishers.

Williams, G. (1984) 'The genesis of chronic illness: narrative re-construction', *Sociology of Health and Illness*, 6(2): 175–200.

Williams, R. (1983) 'Concepts of health: an analysis of lay logic', *Sociology*, 17(2): 185–204.

Williams, S.J. (1995) 'Theorising class, health and lifestyles: can Bourdieu help us?', *Sociology of Health and Illness*, 17(5): 577–630.

Williams, S.J. (1997) 'Modern medicine and the "uncertain body": from corporeality to hyperreality', *Social Science and Medicine*, 45(7): 1041–9.

Williams, S.J. (1998) 'Health as moral performance: ritual transgression and taboo', *Health*, 2(4): 435–57.

Williams, S.J. (2001) 'Sociological imperialism and the profession of medicine revisited', *Sociology of Health and Illness*, 23(2): 135–58.

Williams, S.J. and Calnan, M. (1994) 'Perspectives on prevention: the views of general practitioners', *Sociology of Health and Illness*, 16(3): 372–93.

Williams, S.J. and Calnan, M. (1996) 'The limits of medicalisation: modern medicine and the lay populace in late modernity', *Social Science and Medicine*, 42(12): 1609–20.

Willis, E. (1983) *Medical Dominance*, Sydney: Allen and Unwin.

Willis, E. (1997a) 'The human genome project: a sociology of medical technology', in J. Germov (ed.) *Second Opinion: Sociology of Health and Illness*, Sydney: Oxford University Press.

Willis, E. (1997b) 'Towards healthy public policy: a decade after the Ottawa charter', in *Proceedings of the International Association for Health Policy Conference 1996*, Montreal: University of Montreal.

Wilson, J.D. and Braunwald, E. (1997) *Principles of Internal Medicine*, 14th edn, London: Oxford University Press.

Wilson, P.W., D'Agostino, R.B., Levy, D., Belanger, A.M., Silbershatz, H. and Kannel, W.B. (1998) 'Prediction of coronary heart disease using risk factor categories', *Circulation*, 97: 1837–42.

Wodak, A. (1993) 'HIV infection in drug and alcohol practice', *Medical Journal of Australia*, 158(4): 266.

Wolpe, P.R. (1990) 'The holistic heresy: strategies of ideological challenge in the medical profession', *Social Science and Medicine*, 31(8): 913–23.

Woods, R. (1978) 'Mortality and sanitary conditions in the "Best governed city in the world" – Birmingham 1870–1910', *Journal of Historical Geography*, 4(1): 35–56.

Woodward, J. and Woods, R. (eds) (1984) *Urban Disease and Mortality in Nineteenth Century England*, New York: St Martin's Press.

World Health Organization (1978) *Declaration of Alma Ata*, Regional Office for Europe, Copenhagen: The World Health Organization and the United Nations Children's Fund.

World Health Organization (1985) *Targets for Health for All*, Copenhagen: World Health Organization, Regional Office for Europe.

World Health Organization (1986) *Ottawa Charter*, Copenhagen: World Health Organization, Regional Office for Europe.

Worral, G., Chault, P. and Freake, D. (1997) 'The effects of clinical practice guidelines on patient outcomes in primary healthcare: a systematic review', *Canadian Medical Association Journal*, 156: 1705–12.

Wright, C.M., Parker, L., Lamont, D. and Craft, A.W. (2001) 'Implications of childhood obesity for adult health: findings from thousand families cohort study', *British Medical Journal*, 323: 1280–4.

Wright, P. and Treacher, A. (eds) (1982a) *The Problem of Medical Knowledge: Examining the Social Construction of Medicine*, Edinburgh: Edinburgh University Press.

Wright, P. and Treacher, A. (1982b) 'Introduction', in P. Wright and A. Treacher (eds) *The Problem of Medical Knowledge: Examining the Social Construction of Medicine*, Edinburgh: Edinburgh University Press.

Yeager, K.K., Donehoo, R.S., Macera, C.A., Croft, J.B., Heath, G.W. and Lane, M.J. (1996) 'Health promotion practices among physicians', *American Journal of Preventive Medicine*, 12(4): 238–41.

Zerwic, J.J., King, K.B. and Wlasowicz, G.S. (1997) 'Perceptions of patients with cardiovascular disease about the causes of coronary artery disease', *Heart and Lung*, 26: 92–8.

Zola, K.I. (1972) 'Medicine as an institution of social control', *Sociological Review*, 20(4): 487–504.

Index

Printed in the United States
by Baker & Taylor Publisher Services

Printed in the United States
by Baker & Taylor Publisher Services